52 Years Coping with Chronic... Back Pain

Alvaro Graña

Published by BookPublishingWorld in 2021

Cover Design by Scott Gaunt

Cover Photograph by Alvaro Graña

ISBN: 978-1-8384967-5-3

BookPublishingWorld
is an imprint of
Dolman Scott Ltd
www.dolmanscott.co.uk

Acknowledgements

Most of all, I would like to thank my dear wife Ingrid for her incredible support, understanding and patience during the last 24 years, the most critical period of my life when my condition was deteriorating more and more, both physically and mentally.

I would also like to thank the many doctors, nurses, physiotherapists, and other health professionals, who have helped me over the last 52 years since my sports injury. I would particularly like to show my appreciation and gratitude to Mr. Robert Hatfield, my chiropractor, without whom my life for the last 30 years would have been very different and much more difficult.

I wish to express my love and gratitude to Ingrid, who has spent a lot of time proof-reading my book, and for her patience and understanding, while I have been engaged in writing this book.

I hope many people will find this book helpful, but if it helps just one person in similar circumstances, that would be my greatest wish fulfilled.

THIS BOOK IS DEDICATED TO MY FAMILY.

I dedicate this book to my wife Ingrid, who is my rock, who always supports me in whatever I do, and to the rest of my family, my chidren Natalia and Orlando as well as my grandchildren Maya, Alfie, Javie and River. I hope that one day they will read my book and learn that though there may be problems and suffering in life we each need to face them not as problems but as challenges. I love you all with all my heart and with all my strength.

Foreword

This is the story of one man's experience and his way of coping with pain over a 52 year journey.

The book reads as if Alvaro Graña is talking to the individual reader, relating his ups and downs, revealing his strengths and weaknesses alike; admitting not taking specialist advice too seriously at times, not persevering or giving up, demonstrating he and the reader are likely to have much in common. It is only when things become really difficult that he realises that he needs to follow medical advice more rigidly, and in addition take charge of his situation by doing his own investigations to find ways of helping alleviate his situation.

The author could be described as 'the man next door', he has no medical qualifications, and no prior knowledge of alternative/complementary healing methods or medication.

Therefore, this book is an invitation to fellow chronic pain sufferers to accompany him on his journey, a voyage of discovery, as he finds ways of confronting what would otherwise limit his horizons.

Alvaro talks about failures as well as successes, however it is important to remember that some process or method that was not helpful to the author, has indeed helped others, and viceversa.

The aim of this book is to encourage the readers to take charge of their own individual situation, and to find what works best for them, by pointing out shortcuts, describing what is available and what he has found helpful.

You will note that the reader is repeatedly encouraged to seek medical guidance before trying anything new, rather than 'going it alone'.

On a personal note, I find this book very readable while crammed full of helpful tips and information, as well as some interesting anecdotes.

Ingrid Graña
Editor

Table of Contents

INTRODUCTION - ME AND MY BACK PAIN

I am writing this book in the hope that I will be helping people out there in the wide world, with similar problems to mine. I have been suffering with chronic back pain since my sports injury in 1961, later aggravated by arthritis in my joints in 2002.

There are many things I have learnt over the years, which I would like to share with you. Things I wish I had known earlier. But this happens in any scenario. In any case it is important to be positive and look forward.

There are many joint pain and back pain sufferers all over the world. I am one of them. It has been a long journey for me with my Chronic Back Pain caused by an injury to my lower back whilst playing basketball at the age of 16 (year 1961). This sport's injury happened in Lima, Peru, where I was born. After my injury and for quite a while – I will call this period my *first phase* – I was seen by 2 orthopaedic surgeons from the Mayo Clinic, USA who were visiting Lima at the time. Their diagnosis was that I had broken two vertebrae in my lower back. Their prognosis was not good, medical science was not yet advanced enough for them to offer any treatment beyond a referral to a physiotherapist. They said that in the future surgery might be possible. They also warned me that my condition would deteriorate slowly and that in the worse case scenario I might end up in a wheelchair.

My sport's injury happened whilst playing basketball. I was jumping to get the ball at the same time as a player from the opposing team also jumped causing a mid-air collision. I landed awkwardly on my hands and knees, and my opponent landed on my back. A number of people, including my coach, said they heard the sound of my bones cracking, which resulted in a long-lasting injury. During this phase just after the injury and right through the 1960s I was in constant pain. I was prescribed valium, anti-inflammatories and pain killers. The side effects were horrendous. I even became addicted to valium and it took me a long time and great determination to beat the addiction. I was on strong prescribed medication for forty years until I decided to try alternative solutions, which I will cover later.

In 1973 I came to England (London) to pursue post-graduate studies, I was living with chronic pain all down my spine and my right leg in spite of the strong medication. I will expand on this later.

The start of my *second phase* was when I decided to look into my condition in greater detail, though I still did not grasp the seriousness of my injury.

My advice would be not to leave it all to your doctor, take action, be pro-active and find out as much about your condition as

possible. Speak to other health professionals, search books and the internet, and listen to other people who have experienced pain themselves and have discovered coping mechanisms.

From now on my personal experiences will be in bold and in a different font.

JOINT AND BACK PAIN

Joint and back pain account for a very high percentage of the pain experienced in the world. Joint and back pain can be under the umbrella heading of Musculoskeletal Pain. Symptoms can range from muscular spasms to inflammed joints. Nerve pain can also be experienced and it is characterised by aching – felt sometimes like an electric sensation (an electric current) running up your nerve, and a tingling sensation (a feeling of edginess). You may feel a stabbing or burning pain as well.

We are talking about pain, so let us address these questions:

- Can we accurately measure the various levels of pain people experience?
- Do we know how the brain works and responds to pain?
- Why is pain tolerated at different intensities by each individual?
- Does gender or age make any difference to how we feel and react to pain?
- What is a pain threshold?
- Can endorphins produced by our bodies be as efficient as a painkiller?

Let's start with what pain is.

How can we define PAIN?

The International Association for Study of Pain (IASP) define pain as:

'An unpleasant sensory and emotional experience which is due to actual or potential tissue damage or which is expressed in terms of such damage'.

Pain works as the natural warning system. It is a message sent from any part of the body to the brain (the mind) through our nervous system, to tell us that something is wrong.

Pain can be broken down into the following categories.

Types of pain

Acute Pain: The term 'acute' indicates a relatively abrupt onset with evident symptoms and limited duration. This can be caused by a physical event such as a fall, a sprain or break, as well as an inflammation or infection. Acute pain normally resolves itself as healing occurs.

Chronic Pain: This is long-term pain, unlike acute pain, which is normally temporary and disappears with time and treatment. Chronic pain persists after healing has occurred. Chronic pain is constant and nagging. There are many conditions which produce chronic pain including arthritis, gout, joint pain, and back ache, among others. This type of pain may be either constant or sporadic. It may be difficult to identify its cause.

Referred Pain: Referred pain is felt some distance away from its origin. Osteoarthritis of the hip, for instance, causes pain in the knee.

It is extremely important to seek professional medical advice if your pain persists or has no obvious cause.

Emotional pain: Pain is usually thought as physical, though emotional pain or mental distress can manifest itself in the body. This type of pain can be caused by being rejected, from bereavement, from problems with relationships, etc. One acute form of emotional or psychological distress is depression, a term that covers anything from feeling down and sad to extreme mental and emotional agony. Emotional or mental pain can manifest physically as a headache/migraine, stomach upset, ulcers or even muscle pain (through tension and stress) for example. The causes of these pains can include nightmares, fears, phobias, obsessions, and addictions to food, drink, drugs, etc.

It is important to recognise that long-term emotional pain can lead to physical symptoms as well as the other way around.

Words to do with pain

Describing pain can be very difficult. Here is a list of words that might be associated with pain:

Ache – Anguish – Misery – Suffering – Torture – Affliction – Agony – Discomfort – Pangs – Twinge – Distress – Torment – Wretchedness

How would you describe your pain? These are some symptoms:

You might feel:

- a sharp pain
- a nagging pain
- a persistent/constant pain
- edgy (ie.: nerve pain)
- a stabbing pain
- a niggling pain
- a tight (stiffnes) pain

Pain can result in the following side effects:

- stomach ache
- constipation
- insomnia (difficulties in sleep)
- nausea
- dizziness
- lethargic/spaced out
- very low in energy/tired/exhausted

Describing your mood while carrying pain can also be difficult. These are some descriptions:

- Fed up
- Worried
- Anxious
- Confused
- Depressed
- Angry
- Embarrassed

- Very sad from feeling sorry for yourself
- Frustrated
- Introverted
- Aggressive
- Moody
- Impatient

Other nagging thoughts can be:

- Will the pain stop?
- Financial worries
- Will I lose my job?
- Sexual problems
- I am always loosing my temper
- Why me…?
- I used to be very strong and independent, now look…?
- What will other people think of me? Look at me…
- Will I end up… severely damaged?
in a wheel chair?
being rejected?
- Self-pity

Personal experince - I reacted to pain very badly with a negative response. I got very angry, had mood swings sometimes feeling sorry for myself allowing the pain to get me down. Right through my *first phase* I suffered from regular migrains, which were sometimes severe. I was not in control. In the *second phase* I began to realise how my mental state affected me physically. Talking about nagging thoughts, I experienced most of those mentioned above, including the thought of ending up in a wheelchair in the future, as mentioned

by the doctor I first saw right after my injury. This could be described as the *poor me syndrome.* To summarise, right through my first phase (40 years, from 1961 till 2001) I suffered from regular lower back pain, pain to my sciatic nerve down my right leg, pain to my upper back and migrains. By 2001, I realised that I needed to be more self-aware and to devise a method of how to respond to pain, in order to feel in control of my situation.

How we respond to pain

It is difficult to establish why one person appears to feel less pain than another in similar circumstances. Pain perception is more likely to stem from a combination of factors which may include:

- the state of the individual person's nervous system: This could be due to genetic make-up and/or degenerative consequences. Some people's nervous system is naturally more efficient.
- the consequences of reducing health: Younger people are usually better able to deal with trivial injuries than the majority of older people. In addition to the general effects of ageing, some people become weakened further by chronic disabling illnesses or injuries.
- personality: Where people are of similar age and comparable health, inherent personality may be a motivating factor. People with strong will power, often try harder to conceal what they perceive as deficiencies, whereas other people tend to be more sensitive and less likely to disguise their feelings.
- circumstances: In extreme conditions a person with a focussed mind is often capable of blocking out unpleasant stimuli. An example of this is when soldiers in battle continue to fulfill their mission

despite severe injuries, because of their overriding struggle to win and their survival instinct masks everything else.

Physical pain and psychological pain are very much linked together. One can affect the other. Many medical practitioners, both alternative and conventional are considering a wholistic approach as a more effective form of healing. This means mind and body being treated as a whole rather than as separate entities: the mind can heal the body and the body can heal the mind. For instance using a treatment of diet and exercise, and in addition adopting a positive mental attitude towards his/her living and working conditions, may diminish the symptoms of mental or emotional pain.

Our attitude to pain is absolutely crucial. A negative attitude may lead to extra tension, stress and unhelpful messages being sent from the mind to the body, which consequently aggravate the on-going pain situation. We need to accept pain and work with it, especially those who suffer from chronic pain. The ability to control our reactions, the response of those around us and the situation causing the pain will affect our tolerance to it. Knowledge and understanding could help towards our ability to implement Pain Management.

Personal experience - During my *second phase* I was not mentally strong enough to deal with chronic pain. My negative attitude did not help. I was not in complete control of my stressful life either. I began to realise that I had to juggle lots of things at the same time. Lets go back a bit, between 1973 and 1975, while I was a post-graduate student in London, I started to try different alternative solutions.

My GP referred me to St. Thomas' Hospital. At first they tried Traction Treatment, which included some traction exercises for me to do at home. This was not successful. The doctors then tried epidural injections which were also ineffective. After these unsuccesful treatments they recommnded acupuncture which unfortunately did not help either.

Later I went to see a back specialist at East London Hospital. After a thorough examination and looking at my past history, he recommended specific physio exercises in order to strengthen my back muscles, rather than surgical intervention. At this point I was still hoping for a magical medical cure. Exercise did not seem to me to be a proper medical solution.

During these two years in London, I was not often in control of my pains and mental state. When I practiced *pain management* I was more in control of my life in general, while at other times, when I allowed pain to take over, the pain was more intense. It is possible to endure chronic pain without being controlled by it. It is a matter of knowing how to minimise the pain, knowing that "pain can be let in the gate", as the scientists Melzack and Wall found out.

CHRONIC PAIN - THE GATE CONTROL THEORY OF PAIN

In 1965 two scientists, Ronald Melzack and Patrick Wall, carried out research into pain systems. They proposed that the Gate Control Theory of Pain offers a physiological explanation for the previously observed psychological effects of pain perception.

According to this theory there are '*gates*' in the neuromuscular junctions, the spinal chord and the pain centres in the brain. When these *gates* open and let the message through the system, we feel pain. The *gates* can also stop messages entering the system, so that the pain is reduced or not felt.

In the 1970s, it was discovered that the body can make its own opioid-like substances called endorphins (we shall expand on this later on), which can reduce pain by acting as a pain-killer. Codeine and morphine for instance contain pain relief substances found in opium poppy seeds. Morphine attaches to the same receptors in the brain as endorphins. Endorphins can help close the *gate*. Researches believe that the body releases increased levels of endorphins into the blood stream during and immediately after exercise. These endorphins became the popular answer to anything that gave pleasure, such as regular sex, masturbation and orgasms (more on this later on).

As most chronic pain sufferers know, there are no treatments that can eliminate pain completely. However, according to the Gate Control Theory there are other ways to close the *gate, for example:*

- Pain relief medication
- Physical activity – walking, playing a garden game, swimming, etc
- Pacing activities – doing 'something' in stages
- Relaxation – meditation, slow deep breathing, relax tense muscles, etc
- Distraction – playing a board game (ie,: chess, cards, etc.), engaging in a hobby (painting, drawing, etc), watching a good film, etc
- Addressing stress and worries
- Sitting in a jaccuzi
- Having a warm shower
- Talking to a friend
- Reading a good book
- Interacting with other people – socialising
- Being positive and optimistic

More on these later on.

What opens the *gate*?

- Worry and stress
- Being moody and bad tempered
- Feeling fed-up
- Feeling down
- Moaning and getting angry
- Not enough sleep

- Staying in one position too long
- Getting frustrated
- Being bored and not enjoying life
- Focusing on the pain - Going round in circles thinking about the pain
- Thinking 'why me' and feeling sorry for yourself
- Being negative

Personal experience - In the late seventies and all through the eighties my constant chronic pain continued to increase. My condition was going from bad to worse as I wasn't doing anything about it. I had not taken on board anything I had learnt and I started having severe pains down my legs (especially my right leg). In 1988, by which time I had moved to Coventry, my condition was so bad that I went to see an orthopaedic Surgeon who recommended an operation to my lower back, to which I agreed because I could hardly walk 100 yards without having to stop for a rest. The consultant warned me about the odds: there was a 65% chance that I might end up the same or worse vs a 35% chance that I might find some unquantifiable benefit. I felt I had nothing to lose, so agreed to have the operation. The procedure was a fusion of two vertebrae (L5 and S1).

I was doing voluntary work at the time alongside looking after my 8 year-old daughter and my 4 year-old son. By then I was aware that stress affected my physical condition and aggravated my pain. I felt I was on a vicious downward spiral.

Vicious Spiral of Chronic Pain

As physical and psychological pain are very much linked together, here is a sequence of a possible downward spiral of chronic pain.

The BODY Persistent physical Pain	less active)))))))))))))))))) stiffness, more pain	**The MIND** moody bad tempered	loss of fitness))))))))))))))))))))) weak muscles & joints	
The BODY More physical Pain	lack of energy)))))))))))))) tiredness	**The MIND** worry	stress, fear)))))))))))))) anxiety	**The BODY** even more pain))))))
even less active)))))))))))))))) anger, frustration	**The MIND** you are thinking the worst	negative thoughts))))))))))))))))) fears about the pain	**The BODY** referred pain, other pain	total inactivity)))))))))))))) weaker muscles
The MIND You are desperate Stressed out	depression)))))))))))))))))) isolation	**The BODY** **in a bad way**	concern for future, problems:))))))))))))))))))))))))))))) money, work, relationships, etc	

In this scenario the situation goes from bad to worse to completely out of control. It is a spiral rather than a circle. The aim must be to avoid getting into this downward spiral of pain.

Peronal experience – After my operation I had to spend 6 months convalescing at home with some physiotherapy and rest, gradually returning to a level of normality.

A year after my operation, I did a teacher training - PGCE course at Warwick University, which I completed in spite of my intense physical discomfort. The operation put me back to work, I got

a job as a primary school teacher almost straight away so this might be perceived as a success story.

When I started teaching (1989-90) at Hearsall Community Primary School I did not take any medication other than paracetamol when required, but I found it very tough going. The work was both physically and mentally very demanding which resulted in constant lower back pains, and migraines and neck aches at times.

After my probationary year as a teacher I realised I needed further help with my condition. A friend recommended a chiropractor, whom I went to see (1991). After a few visits I began to notice my condition improving thanks to the treatment. I was going to my chiropractor every week to begin with, then booking appointments as and when necessary and was able to keep the pain under control for the rest of that year.

After a few years my marriage began to crumble adding another level of stress in my life, in addition to the stress from work. It eventually started to affect me physically and mentally and pain once again became more frequent and severe. My marriage ended in divorce, a very painful process. I continued in my determination not to take strong medication for a few more years until one day in 1999 while I was at work teaching 6-7 year-olds, sitting along side my pupils on a very small chair at an equally small table. At the end of the lesson I could not stand up, on a second attempt I felt a horrendous pain on my back and right leg and was unable to move. I was taken to the staff room by some of my colleagues

but as I did not recover I was sent home. This was my darkest hour. Not even my chiro-practor could put me right this time, as he had done previously. I was unable to go back to work for the rest of that year and was on sick pay until it eventually became clear I had to retire on medical grounds in the year 2000.

After I retirerd on medical grounds I decided the time had come for me to take control and started the process of searching and learning more about my condition. It was during that year that I went back to my GP and agreed to try medication again. At the beginning I was dreading it, because of my negative experience with prescribed drugs in Peru between 1967 and 1970 , but felt I had no other option. I hoped medicine would have advanced and was relieved to discover that doctors no longer prescribe valium for chronic pain. I was prescribed painkillers, anti-inflammatories and antidepressants which helped aleviate the pains, but the side effects were horrible. This was the beginning of my *third phase*, a very dark phase. I started finding out about the different types of medication to manage chronic pain and avoid side effects.

Types of Medicine to manage Chronic Pain

There are four types of medicine available:

1. Analgesics: these are commonly known as 'painkillers', such as paracetamol, codeine, tramadol, morphine, among others. Chronic pain sufferers will testify that these drugs can help to reduce pain but do not relieve it completely, while producing side effects which can cause discomfort or pain, for example: constipation, itching,

loss of concentration, nausea, dry mouth, mood changes, problems with sleep, to name but a few.

2. Anti-inflammatories: are used to reduce inflammation and pain in acute pain similar to that caused by a twisted ankle, and chronic pain such as in arthritis. The most commonly used anti-inflammatories are: ibuprofen, indomethacin and diclofenac, which are known as non-steroidal anti-inflammatory drugs (NSAIDs). Unfortunately these may also produce side effects such as: weakness and fatigue, dizziness, flu-like illness, diarrhoea, indigestion, stomach pain, heartburn, nausea, headache, bleeding from the gut, stomach or bowel.
3. Antidepressants: Drugs such as amitriptyline and imipramine are normally used to treat depression. Recent research shows they are also effective in reducing pain and pain-related sleep problems. The amitriptyline dose recommended to manage chronic pain is quite small, 5mg-25mg. Whereas a much higher dose, 100mg-200mg is used for treating depression. Amitriptyline may produce the side effects such as dizziness, constipation, stomach aches, blurred vision, poor concentration, dry mouth.
4. Anticonvulsants: These are used to deal with chronic pain, to treat epilepsy, and also to reduce pain coming from nerve fibres. The most common side effects are nausea and vomiting, dizziness, drowsiness, skin rashes, unsteadiness, and stomach aches. Nowadays the medical profession does not recommend the use of tranquilizers or muscle/mind relaxants, such as diazepam (vallium) for chronic pain as they often lead to dependency (addiction).

If you are using any of the above drugs it is important to report all the side effects, both physical and emotional to your doctor.

Personal experience - My symptoms the year after I stopped working and before I retired on medical grounds were: chronic arthritic type pains to the joints of my spine and legs which affected the nerves, causing inflammation. This inflammation caused various degrees of pain which sometimes affected one, two or more areas of my body (lower back, upper back, neck, right hip joint and knees mainly). The pain occasionally affected my whole body when the inflammation was generalised, which means I was experiencing constant pain of various degrees of intensity.

I sometimes felt dizzy due to severe inflammation and had to lie down in the dark room for hours, and in some instances days at a time. I was prescribed migrain tablets, but they didn't work. Occasionally when the pain was located in a particular area of my spine, it was so intense it caused nausea and vomiting (although it is not clear whether the nausea was caused by the medication or by migrains). I also had occasional pains to my liver, middle back, leg, neck, eyes and head which also induced dizziness and nausea, some times causing vomiting, which I later found out through my chiropractor were migrain symptoms and related to my lower back injury. Sometimes the pains went from the back of my head down my spine, down along my right leg all the way to my heel. It felt like an electric shock travelling from one point to the other.

Later, around 2002, I also had arthritic type pains which started with my hands then progressed to my knees and then to my ankles. My doctor said it was degeneration of the joints (wear and tear) partly to do with my age and partly to do with my injury and the operation. I went for a second opinion and was told it was arthritis. I didn't do much for a whole year when I stopped working and was beginning to get depressed and fed up. Then I don't know what the trigger was, but I decided I was going to do something, I wanted to be active. After some searching, Ingrid my wife who was working full time, I decided to run a business from home (2001). It meant a lot of physical work but I did it. Ingrid supported me from the start helping whenever she had time, though the lion's share fell to me. It was very tough, and I suffered quite a lot of physical setbacks and pain but I realised the pains that I experienced when I was active were about the same as the ones I had when I had been inactive. At least I had an interest, I was active and devised coping strategies and learnt to pace myself. The activity gave me something constructive to focus on, distracting me from my pain, and I was once again a functioning individual, which boosted my morale.

There are two Types of Sufferers

One type is the person who avoids activity and the second type is the person who copes and keeps active.

The avoider:
- gets frightened by the pain and worries a lot about the future.
- is afraid that pain always means further damage, which is not necessarily the case.
- rests a lot and waits, hoping that the pain will diminish or possibly disappear altogether.

The coper:
- knows that the pain will ease and does not fear the future
- carries on as normally as possible.
- deals with the pain by being positive and staying active.

The coper manages by practising PAIN MANAGEMENT.

PAIN MANAGEMENT

Pain Management is learning ways to cope with pain by finding out (knowledge) as much as possible about the origins, causes, treatments; discovering things to avoid, positive attitude, etc, that might help him/her to be in control and manage their pain.

Knowledge leads to understanding which consequently leads to Effective Management. Pain management is recommended to sufferers of chronic, persistent pain.

In the last 20 years hospitals all over Britain have set up 'Pain Clinics' staffed by specialists who deal with people with many different problems who all have one thing in common – persistent or chronic pain. Their main aim is to help people to manage or cope better by understandig more about their pain.

Dr.Tom Smith, in his book "Overcoming Back Pain" (2003), makes a comment about Pain Clinics, "Many of the people attending Pain Clinics have chronic low back pain, - a measure of how ineffective we GPs and orthopaedic surgeons are in treating them. So where are we going wrong?"

EDUCATION plays a very important role in pain management. By practitioners giving a full explanation of the physical and psychological factors which contribute to an individual's pain. From education comes knowledge which leads to understanding; knowledge and understanding empowers the individual to practice pain management

Knowledge + Understanding = MANAGEMENT

Dr. Smith makes reference to cognitive therapy and psychophysiology, two approaches which Pain Clinics around the country use alongside other treatments.

Cognitive Therapy

Cognitive means understanding, so cognitive therapy is learning about pain and how the sufferer can best cope with it. The therapist discusses issues related to pain, fears and beliefs about pain, different treatments, mental attitudes to pain, perceptions of chronic pain, expectations on treatments, confidence, etc. As a result of this learning experience patients can develop their own expertise in dealing with their own pain getting stronger mentally as a result. The patient learns how to avoid dwelling on their pain and realises that stress makes pain worse.

Psychophysiology

Psycho means mind, and physio means body, so it is about how the mind and everything that happens in there affects the body. Our moods, thoughts and feelings have the power to alter physiological reactions in the body. So psychophysiology aims at changing the interaction between the mind and the body, sometimes by simply focussing on something else distracts the pain. The five main tools to be in control of pain are:

1.– Control of breathing
2.– Relaxation
3.– Self-hypnosis
4.– Biofeedback
5.– Meditation

For all these different approaches, please go to section 'The Way Forward – Treatments and Recommendations' (page 28).

These techniques should not be taken lightly. Please be aware that not all will suit everyone, although there should be something for everyone in this 'menu'.

Dr. Smith says, "When we are in pain, we breathe faster and less deeply: if this continues, we pitch into a panic reaction. Understanding how to control and slow down our breathing is critical: by doing so, we slow down all our heightened bodily activities, and our pain perception is lessened." This is something anybody can learn and do. Most Pain Clinics and elementary yoga classes teach breathing techniques as well as meditation.

All techniques are explained in most Pain Clinics, and you will be made aware that they require focus, dedication and time; perseverance will pay off, they are not a quick fix. Ensure to always seek professional advice.

Personal experience - After I became more active in the third phase I started to work out what I could do without aggravating my condition and also the things I needed to avoid doing. The most important goal I set myself was to try and live life as normally as possible and focus on the things I could do rather than the things I couldn't do. I also learnt to stop and take time to rest and recover for the next stint. By trial and error I learnt about the things and activities that I should avoid. It was all about awareness and management.

THINGS THAT YOU CAN DO FOR YOURSELF

There are various actions you can take to help yourself.

You can:

- live life as normally as possible.
- keep up your daily activities avoiding heavy lifting/activity
- try to get fit by walking, swimming, or specific exercises (see Section PHYSICAL EXERCISES (page 58) on a regular basis.
- Stop any worries, and tensing up, to avoid feeling down or even depressed.
- Use relaxation techniques to avoid stress.(see RELAXATION page 149)
- Pace yourself - do a bit at a time, increasing your level of activity as time goes on. Monitor your activity to see clearly how you are coping. (see PACING – page 82).
- Be patient when looking for results and give yourself time.
- Be positive and realistic. A positive mind will give you a positive attitude, which will make you more active, able to resume normal activity giving you a sense of achievement and that all round feel-good effect, which will have a positive influence on your body. Remember not to over do it. (see POSITIVE MENTAL ATTITUDE – page 74)
- Stay as active as you can.

– Maintain general good health. (See GOOD GENERAL HEALTH (page 88).

THINGS TO AVOID

- Heavy lifting – lift what you can handle – always lift close to your body – bend your knees and no stooping, let your legs do the work for you – avoid twisting your back.
- Sitting in one position for a long time – use a support if necessary – use an upright chair – if after a while you feel stiff, get up and stretch.
- Standing still for a long time.
- Staying in bed for a long time, but if it is inevitable, try gentle stretching and joint movement excersises– stretch before going to sleep and before you get up in the morning.
- Feeling negative and disgruntled when you are in pain or experiencing low energy – tell yourself 'this is only temporary' and plan the next step for as soon as you are able to be active; this will give you something to focus on, keep you in a positive frame of mind and give you something to look forward to.

Personal experience – Due to a series of unexpected and unavoidable chain of events I was living with very high stress levels and realized this was detrimental to my condition. In my effort to bring my stress level down I was trying to live as normally as possible after concluding that, come what may, I am responsible for my own wellbeing. If I am in pain I have to be proactive and take action. I have to analise the scenario and work out why I

am in pain. Is it something physical? Something I have done? Or is it something mental/psychological? Stress maybe? I began to notice that whenever I was in a lot of pain and exhausted, I was also feeling down, had negative thoughts, and was sometimes in a bad mood. I eventually realised that this was to do with my mental attitude and my reaction to pain...perhaps focusing too much on it. I decided I had to change my attitude.

PAIN SUFFERING SCENARIOS

There are at least three pain suffering scenarios pain sufferers might find themselves in:

Scenario 1 - Suffering from pain and taking no action other than relying heavily on prescribed medication resulting in having no confidence.

Scenario 2 - Suffering from pain and taking some action as well as taking prescribed medication. This action may involve trying complementary medicine in negligible quantities, too little to be of any benefit, expecting instant results and not giving it enough time to take effect.

Another action might be doing specific exercises to help with the pain, but in a controlled manner: pacing yourself, building it up slowly, and efficiently so that the muscles and ligaments do not get strained or damaged.

Maybe trying a different alternative treatment, once again not taking it very seriously, as lack of confidence brings doubt.

Scenario 3 - Suffering from pain and taking positive action. Taking everything seriously, in a controlled manner, maximising efficiency. For instance deciding to take up complementary medicine, taking the recommended daily amounts on a regular basis. Deciding to try exercises and conscienciously following expert advice in a controlled manner, pacing yourself to maximise efficiency. Self discipline and persistence will result in reaching good fitness levels.

Analogy: One might be able to run around the block now and again in spite of not being fit, however a daily run of increasing length will result in fitness.

Looking into alternative solutions and staying positive will accomplish good results and boost confidence.

Personal experience - After a few years of trying really hard to live a normal life with the help of prescribed medication, remaining as active as I could by being pro-active in dealing with pain, and trying hard to have a positive attitude to chronic pain, I learnt various tips, such as pacing myself, avoiding lifting heavy things, not bending my back and avoiding stress among other things. I was still determined to find new solutions: I wanted to give up prescribed medication, so I went to see my GP (2003) who referred me to a Qualified Alternative Medicine Practitioner at University Hospital in Coventry. At that point I was suffering from joint pains everywhere, in addition to my usual pains to my lower back, neck and legs. Every morning I would wake up with pain in my joints (feet, ankles, knees, hips, elbows and hands). More on this later.

So in summary, my condition has always been twofold: nerve pains in my spine from the back of my head down to my heels affecting two or more areas of my body, caused by inflammation to the nervous system. I sometimes experienced referred pains (inflammation) to my liver and other internal organs. This happens because nerves coming from the spine are connected to internal organs. I also suffered from severe migraines, sciatic pains in my leg (especially my right leg), and inflammation to the joints in my hip. When the inflammation affected my coxis, I found sitting very painful.

By this time I was slowly learning how to live with this condition which meant carrying various degrees of pain, being unable to move at times but still maintaining a positive attitude and a cool head to avoid depression.

CAUSES OF JOINT PAIN

Joint pain can be caused by many types of injuries or conditions. The following are some of the most common ones:

- Unusual exertion – A strain or sprain the ligaments or muscles can result from a sudden movement, improper movement or through overuse. In the case of back pain, discs can be damaged in the same way, and they can tear or overstretch.
- Injury, including fracture
- Osteoarthritis is the most common form of Arthritis. This chronic disease causes the cartilage between the bone joints to wear away, leading to stiffness and pain. OA, as it is known, involves growth of bone spurs and degeneration of cartilage at a joint (common in adults over the age of 45).
- Septic arthritis, which is the inflammation to a joint caused by bacterial invasion.
- Tendonitis, which is the inflammation, irritation and swelling of a tendon which is the fibrous structure that connects muscle to bone.
- Bursitis, which is inflammation to the bursa that lies between a tendon and skin or between a tendon and bone. The bursae are fluid filled sacs that cushion and pad bones allowing muscles and ligaments to move freely.
- Gout, which is specially found in the big toe.

- Infectious diseases can include the following:
  - Influenza
  - Measles
  - Rheumatic fever
  - Hepatitis
  - Mumps
  - Rubella (German Measles)
  - Varicela (Chicken Pox)
  - Osteomyelitis
- Auto immune diseases, such as rheumatoid arthritis and lupus.

Arthritis

Arthritis is inflammation of one or more joints, which results in pain, swelling and limited movement. Arthritis involves the breakdown of the cartilage which normally protects the joint, allowing for smooth movement. Cartilage also absorbs shock when pressure is placed on a joint while walking, running or jumping. Without the usual amount of cartilage, the bones rub together, causing pain, swelling (inflammation) and stiffness.

Osteoarthritis

This type of arthritis is usually caused by a mechanical failure in the joint, with changes occurring in the articulate cartilage and bone. OA is a degenerative disease which most commonly affects the hip, knee, spine and finger joints. There are three main causes of osteoarthritis:

1. wear and tear as a result of the ageing process
2. as a result of an injury or surgical intervention
3. abnormal weight bearing placed on joints (especially hips and knees) over a considerable period of time or as a result of long-term obesity.

Rheumatoid Arthritis

This type of arthritis is caused mainly by chronic inflammation in the synovial linings of joints, tendon sheaths and bursae (sacs of fibrous tissues containing synovial fluid). The synovial lining coats the inside of the joint structure and produces fluid to help lubricate joint movement.

Ankylosing Spondylitis

Spondylitis means inflammation in the joints linking the vertebrae in the spinal cord. In ankylosing spondylitis the acute inflammation has receded leaving toughened damaged joints that have become fused together causing pain and restricted movement of the spine.

Joint Inflammation

Causes of joint inflammation include:

- broken bones
- infection (usually caused by bacteria or viruses)
- an auto immune disease
- general wear and tear on joints. Most of the time inflammation

resolves after an injury has healed, although in some cases, the inflammation persists, becoming long-term (chronic) and deformity occurs. This is refered to as chronic arthritis. Osteoarthritis is the most common type and is more likely to occur as part of the aging process.

Symptoms

May include:

- Joint pain
- Joint swelling
- Stiffness, especially in the morning
- Sensation of warmth around the joint
- Redness of the skin around the joint
- Reduced ability to move the joint.

Personal experience - The Alternative Medicine Specialist recommended me to take *glucosamine sulphate* and *evening primrose oil* together. She told me three important steps I needed to take:

1. **She said according to research the dose recommended for me is 1500 mgs of each, daily.**
2. **Allow a long period of time before expecting the full effect (2 to 3 months maybe).**
3. **I had to carry on taking my prescribed medication and slowly reducing it over at least 2 or 3 months until I could stop it altogether.**

This is what I did, under medical supervision, and it worked. When I say it worked, I mean that although not all the pains disappeared, I managed to not depend on prescribed medication, consequently avoiding all the side effects. This process took approximately 6 to 8 months. After a year I went to see the Alternative Medicine Specialist again and she said that according to new research in America and Canada, they found out that the normal dose mentioned above, when doubled, was even more effective. It was safe to increase the dose because they are all natural ingredients rather than drugs, and I had not shown any adverse reaction. People who are going to try this need to consult their doctor and make sure you are not allergic to shell fish (in the case of glucosamine sulphate) or any other component.

I increased both the evening primrose oil and the glucosamine sulphate to 3000mgs a day. It took a few months before I started to feel the benefits. My arthritic type pains in my knees, ankles, elbows and hands were almost gone (2006-07). Remember I said, I used to wake up every morning with terrible joint pains and found getting up a struggle? I don't any more. Even the pain to my elbow is gone. This might be to do with the fact that I am a musician, and play quite a few string instruments. It is now about 14 years since I had serious pains in the mornings which made it difficult to get out of bed. The other recommendations that I received from the specialist was to do exercises guided by a physiotherapist, and eat a healthy diet. More on these last two points and complementary medicine later.

Treatment

Not all cases are curable.

Some recommendations:

- making lifestyle changes
- Pacing yourself – although it is good to keep busy and active, pacing yourself should be part of the new lifestyle. Only you know how much you can do and still feel positive (see more below).
- Exercise to maintain healthy joints, relieve stiffness, reduce pain and fatigue, improve muscle tone and bone strength. Exercise programmes need to be designed by a professional as an individualised programme according to each condition.
- Cold and heat treatment as needed – bearing in mind that muscles need heat, while nerve inflammation needs cold. Try both and see what works as it is sometimes difficult to pinpoint the origin of pain.
- Rest and exercise are both important, again try both and see what helps. It is sometimes helpful to take naps or lie down during the day, to recover from a flare-up more quickly. If you need a longer rest, bear in mind that this is temporary. To stay positive think and plan what you will be doing next.
- Avoid positions or movements that place extra stress on your affected joints.
- Avoid holding one position for too long.
- Reduce stress, avoid worrying about things and tensing up, or stress from work as these can aggravate symptoms. Try to relax by using meditation, guided imagery, yoga or Tai Chi, on these last two consult your doctor.
- Modify your home if it is going to make your life easier.

- Taking glucosamine sulphate and evening primrose oil in combination (always consult your doctor first) – They don't work for everybody with joint or back pain, but they are worth a try.
- Healthy eating – Eat sensibly and avoid becoming overweight to minimise the pressure on your joints. Take calcium to keep your bones strong (around 700 to 1000mg a day) by eating dairy products, small boned fish, fortified bread and cereals, or calcium supplements (always consult your doctor first). Eat a diet rich in vitamins and minerals, especially antioxidants like vitamin E. These are found in fruit and vegetables. Brewer's yeast, wheat germ, garlic, whole grains, sunflower seeds, and brazil nuts contain selenium. Omega-3, which is shown in studies to reduce inflammation in arthritis and slow the process of joint damage, can be found in fatty acids from cold water fish, (like salmon, mackerel and herring), flaxseed, rapeseed oil, soybeans, soybean oil, pumpkin seeds and walnuts. Therefore the key to keeping healthy joints is regular exercise (see section EXERCISE – page 58) and a healthy diet (see GENERAL HEALTH – page 100).

Personal experience - After my consultation with the Complementary Medicine Specialist at Walsgrave University Hospital I went to see a physiotherapist. I was determined to give exercising on a regular basis a good go. I remember being advised to do this before my operation, but didn't follow it seriously. I did this time. The idea was to strengthen all the muscles around my waist by doing abdominal and lower back exercises; plus stretching and contraction exercises for my legs and body in general. I later added exercises for my neck, which had been one of my weak points for a long time.

My physiotherapist was very supportive and encouraged me to take exercising seriously and consistently. I still remember what she said *"As you brush your teeth everyday, you should do your exercises every day too,"* adding that *"It will take a bit of time before you see any progress."* I followed her advice persevering with the physio exercises and later down the line I was able to see the difference. I still do them today (December 2020). The specialist worked on my physical fitness as well as on my mental attititude by recommending and teaching me the different exercises I need to do every morning before getting up. She advised me to start doing only 5 repeats of each exercise; and very slowly increase the number over a period of time. After four years of slowly increasing the number of some of my exercises, now I do 100 of each as well as my lower back muscle exercises, and 500 abdominal exercises (which I do lying on my back, knees up. I do them in bed before I get up). More on these exercises and how they should be done later. I feel fit and strong now in those areas of my body. Again I am not saying that all my pains have disappeared but I am a lot stronger and my body can cope with pain better. After four or five years following the daily exercise programme I no longer get the regular severe pains on my lower back. When I do ocasionally experience pain, my recovery time is quicker and better. I no longer get any of the strong abdominal pains nor the nausea (I used to feel so sick sometimes that I used to vomit due to the pain). I still had severe pains to my neck and head (similar to severe migraine attacks) occasionally, but today (2020) I hardly get migrains. When I get migrains I use the hot and cold treatment, by putting hot and cold around my neck and shoulders at bed time. I do a bit of relaxation (see relaxation techniques below), which helps me to go to sleep. In 2018 I started having pains in my neck (this time it was different, not migrains) and went to see a physio who recommended exercises for my neck, and now (2020) I am free of pain.

What is most important to acknowledge here is that various different treatments and/or actions can be used to help deal with chronic pain. In fact I would advise everybody to try different methods, without taking any risks, and use those which you find will help in the long run. That is certainly my approach, at present I am using various different treatments and actions simultaneously, and they all help a little. Obviously you are going to use treatments, such as heat and cold packs when in pain at different times alongside regular exercise, a warm wheat bag at bedtime, and a healthy diet. The combination of exercises and the previously mentioned glucosamine sulphate and evening primrose oil are the perfect combination for me. You can oil your joints as you would a squeeky door!

By 2006-07 I had stopped having arthritic type pains.

Another problem I had years ago was pain on my heels when I walked. If I walked 10 or 15 minutes barefoot around the house I would end up with pains on my back and heels. I tried various cushion heel pads which helped a little, then found using two cushion pads in each shoe felt better.

Later, I realised gel cushion pads were the best. I tried layering them...; by 2015 I was using 4 layers of gel cushion heel pads,

2 – 2.5cms. high. The disadvantage is that I can't wear moccasins or sandals any more, but I prefer to minimise my pains.

BACK PAIN

The Anatomy of the back

The back is a complex structure of bones built around the spinal column. The spinal column consists of 24 small bones called vertebrae. There are 7 in the neck (cervical); 12 in the upper back (thoracic) and 5 in the lower back (lumbar). In addition there are 5 fused bones called the sacrum, plus 4 more small bones called the coccyx.

The spinal cord runs through a hole in each of the vertebrae. The nerve roots are attached to the cord, linking them to the brain. The spinal joints are held together by a network of ligaments and a series of faced joints. The bones of the spine are connected to one another by the discs, which act as 'shock absorbers'.

Each joint is surrounded by tough, fibrous muscles and together with the ligaments, keep the back strong.

With such a complex structure, it is not surprising to see so many people suffering from back problems.

Causes of Back Pain

Back pain is one of the most common types of pain. More working days are lost through back problems than any other illness, except flu.

There is not one back problem equal to another, they vary in intensity, the symptoms and causes are different, and referred pain, and emotional pain vary in each individual. The same can be said about joint pain.

The causes of back pain are numerous, among them:

- From an injury, through exertion, lifting, severe blow or fall.
- Straining the ligaments or muscles from a sudden movement, improper movement or through overuse, e.g.: postural strain (improper position when sitting, standing or bending).
- Sprains to ligaments and muscles in the same way.
- From an infection.
- Nerve dysfunction.
- Osteoporosis, tumours.
- Spondylosis (hardening and stiffening of the spinal column)
- Congenital problem
- Childbirth
- Poor diet
- Stress and anxiety
- Damage to discs caused by a sudden or improper movement
- Torn or stretched ligaments

All conditions are different, so always consult your doctor.

Persistent and Chronic Back Pain

If the pain persists over a long time, other events and factors might make it more likely to continue. For instance, if the back muscles become weak, this will reduce the ability of the spine to take further physical stresses. It will become more strenuous to do other activities, and this in turn will compound the problem by affecting the sufferer's confidence and have a detrimental effect on the mind leading to anxiety, frustration, anger and a general negative outlook, which could lead to depression. This can happen to anyone, therefore remembering that both physical and psychological factors can combine to continue to aggravate the pain and create a v*icious spiral of pain* (see Vicious Spiral of Chronic Pain – pg. 16). Also sections "How We Respond to Pain" (pg. 10), and "Types of Pain" (pg. 6).

Stress

This is one of the problems people with chronic pain have to deal with.

The word 'stress' is very popular today. It is commonly used to describe the way we feel when pressure is intense. It is a combination of symptoms produced when our physical, mental and emotional systems go into overdrive. People under stress react differently and get more upset than they would normally do when faced by difficult situations.

High stress levels for people with chronic pain are likely to stem from:
- Unremitting discomfort
- Lack of sleep
- Feeling that you can't have your illness under your control
- Difficult relationships and pressures from other people.
- Lack of knowledge
- Low morale
- Self pity
- Uncertainty about the future

Sources of Stress

Can be both internal and external. Internal can be for instance, a headache; and external can be pressure from your boss or some one else (or a situation). Both internal and external stresses affect our moods, specifically our minds, which consequently affect our physical abilities to cope.

Unfortunately, not all sources of stress are within our control.

There are various stress triggers to be aware of:
- Tiredness caused by insufficient sleep
- Prolonged intense pain
- Feeling fragile, stemming from anger or anxiety
- Frustration and pressures created by others, or by situations
- Discomfort – feeling too cold or too hot
- Feeling isolated – little or no social contact
- Depressing weather

- Work pressures
- Relationship/marriage problems
- Financial problems/debt
- Sensitive digestive system – side effects from long term prescribed medication, or too much alcohol, too much caffeine, etc, which can all exacerbate stress.
- Uncertainty about the future
- Self pity

THE WAY FORWARD – TREATMENTS AND RECOMMENDATIONS

Relying on only one particular solution/treatment, for instance relying on what your doctor has prescribed in terms of pain killers, anti-inflammatories, antidepressants, etc. (which may produce side effects) may not be the only way forward. Try some of the many other options to minimise pain alongside prescriptions, which, if followed sensibly with professional guidance, can lead to little or no pain.

Most of the following treatments and recommendations can be done at the same time with no or very little interference from each other. Every action/treatment/ precaution you take will help to improve your overall well being.

The way forward is to resolve to take personal responsibility for your pain. Consider the following steps:

1. Understanding your condition/illness/pains (as partly covered above).

   Research and learn about your condition/illness/pain as much as pssible. Aim at being an expert on what affects you. This will help in two ways: firstly by providing the knowledge to be able to understand your condition, and secondly by equipping you to discuss the matter with your doctor and work in partnership with them. My advice is to start by finding out about:

- how pain works in your body
- understand the difference between acute and chronic pain
- learn about the physiological processes that are happening, ie. the nervous system and how it processes the information associated with pain by amplifying it
- whether caused by injury, illness or other factors such as an infection, or organ malfunction
- be able to differenciate muscle pain and nerve pain, among others

2. Learn about all the various options/treatments to be practiced as precautions to deal with your particular problem. Although this book concentrates mainly on back and joint pain many of the following options could also be appropriate to other conditions.
3. Resolve to find medical or health professionals with whom you are comfortable, a good doctor, chiropractor, osteopath, therapist, that will listen to you and be willing to work with you as a partner in healing.
4. Resolve to take action on the various options you and your doctor or therapist have decided to try. Be prepared to learn, and flexible to alter the process of implementing the treatments.

POSSIBLE SOLUTIONS - TREATMENTS – ACTIONS

1. Movement and Inactivity

a.- Movement and being active

Pain and movement have a very close relationship capable of affecting each other. Pain causes people to move differently in order to protect the painful area. Incorrect posture, bad habits, and certain movements can also cause pain by stretching muscles and/or overloading joints.

Anyone suffering from ankle pain will limp for a while, reduce their activity and maybe use crutches at the beginning. This allows the injury to recover so healing can take place. This is called **adaptive behaviour**, the person adapts his/her behaviour to suit their condition.

Someone with the same injury might rest the ankle for too long, particularly if worried about making the problem worse, is showing **maladaptive behaviour.** This response is common and understandable from people who suffer spinal pain or chronic pain. Inactivity will inhibit the healing process which consequently leads to joint stiffness, muscle weakness and pain, making the problem worse. It will also cause incorrect movement creating an imbalance in the body, which could lead to reflected pain elsewhere, as well as causing fatigue and stress in the muscles which are working less. This in turn can create more pain in the affected area and new pains elsewhere, perpetuating the process. The solution is to **remain active, without overdoing it!**

Personal experience - This is exactly what happened to me. As mentioned above I had a severe sports injury to my lower back. After I was able to walk again and lead a reasonable normal life (not able to practice sports or streneous activities) my back pain became chronic and constant, becoming worse as time went on. After a long time I started to have pain higher up in the middle of my spine, at the top of my spine (neck) and down my legs (sciatica). These pains also went from bad to worse over a long period of time. My chiropractor explained this was due to the imbalance caused as my body tried to compensate due to the pain of the original injury .

Generally speaking inactivity makes muscles, including the heart, lose strength and work less efficiently. This might possibly lead to increased propensity to high blood pressure, high cholesterol and diabetes. Inactivity can also increase fatigue, stress and anxiety, **which I have experienced in the past.**

Inactivity breeds inactivity, the less you do, the less you feel like doing, aggravating the situation. Exercise can be a great solution to ease chronic back pain, but always consult your doctor or physiotherapist first.

b.- The benefits of movement

Movement, activity and exercise helps the body:

- to strengthen muscles and ligaments
- to increase flexibility
- to improve sleep quality
- to boost energy levels
- to maintain a healthy weight
- to enhance mood
- to protect heart and blood vessels
- to release endorphines (see Activating Endorphines (page 107)

Note: All the above is advice given to patients at the Mayo Clinic in the USA.

c.- Movement and blood circulation.

Movement is essential to maintain good circulation, particularly drainage of blood. When someone is in pain, he/she moves less, and the part that moves less has poor circulation. The damage to tissues is usually the tearing muscle, ligament or disc fibres. Tissue damage very often results in inflammation, which can be very painful.

We need to say it again, too much rest hoping for the pain to go away results in poor circulation, so move around as much as you can in a sensible way. Muscle spasm can be painful and slow down the flow of blood (circulation) and other tissue fluids.

d.- Physical Exercise

Any good exercise programme should achieve three things:

- flexibility
- strengthening
- endurance
- If your back is not flexible, you are more likely to overstretch something.
- If your back is not strong, you are more likely to strain something.
- If your back tires easily, then you are more likely to strain something.
- Regular exercise in moderation can relieve pain and stiffness.

First and foremost I would like to stress that, from my own experience, EXERSCISE IS THE MOST IMPORTANT ACTION YOU CAN TAKE TO RECOVER FROM A BACK INJURY. But please do not do anything without professional advice and guidance.

Personal experience - As a general principle, people who are fit (without over doing it), suffer less back pain than people who are not fit. Most professionals will tell you that if you are a chronic back pain sufferer, you need to build up your fitness gradually. In the year 2000, when I had already retired, I went to see my physiotherapist for the second time. She recommended to do stretching exercises and to carry on with the other exercises she had previously taught me. I had severe pains on my spine from head to toe. I did my exercises diligently every day, following my physiotherapist instructions and advice.

But I do take a rest when I feel I need it, but not too much. I maintain some level of activity and movement, even when I am not feeling very well, and engage in gentle exercises to keep my back fit and supple. Abdominal muscles are also very important. The abdominal and back muscles work together to hold the trunk upright. That is why my physio encouraged me to do abdominal exercises, starting with a few and slowly building up. I started by doing only ten each day (I still do them every morning as soon as I wake up before getting out of bed). I started with 25-30 repeats and in a year I was doing 100, and 6 months later I was doing 500, which I continue to do. Today (December 2020), I do exercises to ALL my joints, from hands to toes. For some I still do 25/30 repeats, for others I do 50 and 100, and 500 abdominal repeats.

The abdominals are a group of 6 muscles that extend from various parts of the ribs to various parts of the pelvis. They provide movement and support to the trunk, and assist in the breathing process. Sarah Keys says in her "Back Sufferes Bible", "Tummy muscles play a critical role in letting the spine bend. The deepest tummy muscle, transversus abdominus, plays a unique role as it helps the spine straighten, because it works both as a tummy and back muscle at the same time. Practising therapists around the world recognise the importance of a strong tummy in treating back problems". They are possibly **the most used muscles in your whole body.** Try focussing on those muscles when you sit down, or sit up, or run, walk or jump, lie down or sit up after lying down; you will feel how those muscles are working and helping your lower back muscles.

Stretching

To stretch a muscle is to elongate it by moving its ends away from one another. Stretching is generally recommended by doctors, therapists and other professionals to help prevent injury and relieve chronic back pain.

How to go about it: ease into it, start gently, warm up and do not over do it. If you feel any pain when stretching, **stop!** If you feel any pain or are very sore from exercise the following day, it probably means you over did it. Rest for a couple of days, and start again at a lower intensity. If pain and discomfort continues consult your doctor or physiotherapist.

For some people exercise can be very painful, especially at the beginning. I can fully understand why people with joint pains or back pains may want to avoid physical activity. However, remaining sedentary and not moving your joints at all, can compound the problem.

Personal experience - This happened to me when I retired in 2001. I spent a whole year just sitting around doing absolutely nothing at home. I used to wake up every morning with very stiff and painful joints. I could hardly walk, and could hardly move my fingers. The doctor said I had arthritis and prescribed painkillers, which I refused to take. I had taken them for back pain in the past and experienced terrible side effects. So I decided to go to my physiotherapist, and started doing exercises for my joints. Very soon, after only a few weeks, I started to feel the benefits so I carried on, and today I do not have any joint pains. I do have other pains which I manage well (mentioned above), but

currently have neither the stiffness nor the pains in my fingers, wrists, knees or ankles that I had before. By 2007 I was clear of pains in my joints, excluding my lower back. I can manage my back pains very well now, and still suffer from some pain to my lower back but I can live a more or less normal life, albeit with some limitations such as not going for long walks. When I go for a longer walk I take 15-20 minutes' rests as and when my pain tells me I need it, then I am able to carry on walking. Through perseverance I am getting better and better as time goes on.

Please go to Appendix 1 and see "Benefits of Stretching Exercises" (page 145).

So, a well controlled exercise programme can benefit people with arthritis and back pain, helping to avoid pains and prevent injuries. In my case this exercise programme was done in combination with the complementary medicine (evening primrose oil and glucosamine sulphate) previously mentioned. Human joints need oil, like hindges in a door.

Please go to Appendix 2 and see "Arthritis – How to Keep Your Joints Healthy" (page 147).

Posture

Good posture aims to minimize the strain on all the parts of the body, it is a form of fitness in which the muscles of the body support the skeleton in an alignment that is stable and efficient during movement. Good posture is the position in which the different parts of the body are held in such a way as to minimise the strain on all the parts. Unfortunately good posture is not always considered.

– Standing

~ there should be even pressure between the heel and the ball of the foot
~ both knees straight with the knee caps 'loose' not locked
~ shoulders should be back and relaxed
~ head high; neck straight; chin straight (not lifted)

– Sitting

~ bottom should be right at the back of the seat
~ You should have 90 degrees angles at ankles, knees, hips and elbows.

– Lying

~ a good mattress should help support you in a correct position.
~ lumbar spine relaxed, straight and supported by mattress.
~ neck relaxed and supported by pillow
~ body's natural curves supported both when lying on your back or lying on your side.

Personal experience - Choosing a good mattress and a good pillow when your spine is straight and relaxed, and aligned with your neck is essential. It took me a long time to realise this, and it has made a big difference to my quality of sleep.

The most common causes of poor posture are:

– Injury and muscle protection.- After an injury, nearby muscles begin to protect the vulnerable area. These muscles will work in a diminished way to keep the affected part stable and free from injury. This is totally understandable and necessary, but it causes those muscles to weaken.

- Disease and nutritional state.- Deficiencies and disease can negatively affect posture. The presence of disease, dehydration or malnutrition, can cause conditions that directly affect the muscles and bone structures.
- Habit.- People develop bad habits without realising that certain movements they make without thinking affect some part of their bodies.
- Muscle tension, muscle weakness.- If the body has areas that are particularly weak or strong, it will not be held upright in the most effective way which will result in poor posture and pain.
- Mental attitude and stress.- Often stress leads to a decrease in full breathing, which in turn affects body posture, as the two are linked.
- Heredity.- Sometimes bad posture is just in the genes.
- Inappropriate footwear- If one wears down the outside of the shoes faster than the inside, this will create posture imbalance.

The Alexander Technique is a highly recommended plan of action to take in regard to correcting posture. There are many specialists in this field. You could find one either by personal recommendation or by looking on the internet.

e. - Other “structured activities”

Some of the ‘structured activities’ you could try are: yoga, taichi and pilates. This is by no means an exhaustive list. Always consult your medical practicioner before embarking on a new excersise regime.

2. Medication

a.- Traditional Western Medicine.-

This refers to medication prescribed by a doctor in contrast with eastern medicine or complementary/alternative medicine, which will be explained later on.

On page 16 above, I mention the 4 types of medicine frequently prescribed by doctors to manage chronic pain. These are:
1.- analgesics – painkillers
2.- anti-inflammatories
3.- antidepressants
4.- anticonvulsants

Personal experience - I have tried prescribed medication from all 4 types at different points in my life to deal with my chronic back pain, which started in 1961. Right at the beginning, I was taking strong painkillers and a high dosis of valium on a daily basis. I became addicted to valium, as mentioned at the beginning of this book. As addictions go, I felt the need to take valium even though the only thing it did was to suppress the pain. After trying different treatments and medications, in the late 70s, I found none of them were of any major help. My pains carried on, and my general condition deteriorated over the years, until my operation in 1989. This op got me back to work until I had to retire on medical grounds in the year 2000. Between the operation and the return of previous symptoms which led to my retirement I hardly took any medication. I went back to the doctor and started

taking prescribed medication again: strong pain killers, anti-inflammatory tablets(such as diclofenac), antidepressants (such as amitriptyline) and even anticonvulsants (such as Diazepan). They all produced very painful and uncomfortable side effects, although they helped somewhat with the pains. As mentioned above, I eventually gave up all prescribed medication except the amitriptyline, which helped with the pains I had on my neck and the migrains I suffered at the time. Eventually I decided to get advice from a physio to see whether by doing neck exercises, I could get rid of my pains. It worked, so I stopped taking the amitriptyline as well. I am not suggesting that everybody should do this, but this is just one of the actions I took among others, such as exercise taken very seriously (mentioned above), trying alternative medicine (see next point), and other things which I shall cover later on in this section.

b.- Complementary/Alternative Medicine.-

The following are the medicines that the doctor at the hospital recommended to me:

Glucosamine Sulphate, and evening primrose oil, but taking double the recommended dose, as mentioned above. After having double the dose for years (3000mgs each), around 2015, I decided to increase it to 4000mgs each, which is the amount I am taking today (2020).

Before we go on we need to highlight the opinion of a doctor from the Mayo Clinic in the USA.

Dr. Morie Gertz, a hematologist, who chairs the Mayo Clinic's internal medicine department, said: "Most of the doctors here were top of their medical school class, top of their residency, blah,blah,blah, etc. That is technical mastery: that doesn't make them effective healers. Over the past 30 years, I have seen hundreds of patients who clearly feel they have benefited from alternative therapies. It is not my job to tell them they shouldn't feel better, neither to tell them they shouldn't try complemnentary medicine. If they want to, we need to follow the clues patients give us about what might help them. If a patient chooses to walk away from the therapy I have prescribed and go to an alternative therapist instead, that is not the fault of alternative medicine: it is because I have failed as a doctor to do a good job of making my case in terms that are important to the patient".

The above applies to all complementary/alternative medicine we are going to cover below. In my experience, some worked really well, some didn't much and some didn't work at all. I totally agree with Dr. Gertz, when he says that it is up to the patient to feel they are benefiting from alternative medicine or not. Precisely that is my experience.

Glucosamine

Glucosamine aids joint pain and stiffness.

What is glucosamine?

Glucosamine is a molecule made of glucose (sugar) and an amine that is produce naturally in the body.

What is its function?

Glucosamine creates cushioning fluids and tissues around joints.

How does it work in our body?

Glucosamine helps joint function. It stimulates cartilage cells to produce two proteins that help to hold joint tissue together (proteoglycans and collagen), renewing synovial fluids and repairing joints.

How can it help damaged joints?

Research backs the idea that glucosamine can aid in repairing damaged cartilage, building new cartilage, cushioning joints, relieving pain and reducing inflammation.

Is glucosamine naturally produced in the human body?

A certain amount of glucosamine is produced within the body, however bodies lose the capacity to make enough glucosamine as part of ageing, so the cartilage in joints such as the hips, knees and hands is destroyed, it hardens and forms bone spurs which cause pain, deformed joints and limited movement.

How is glucosamine manufactured? Its source?

Glucosamine supplements are manufactured from chitin, a substance (a carbohydrate), formed in shrimp, crab and lobster shells.

Are there any side effects?

The most common side effects are increased intestinal gas and softened stools. Other possible side effects are bloating, constipation, heartburn, nausea and stomach upset. Other more unusual side effects are drowsiness, skin reactions, vomiting, headache, elevated blood pressure and heart rate, and palpitations.

Check with your doctor as some people may be allergic to shellfish and should therefore avoid glucosamine altogether, unless it has been confirmed that it is from a non-shellfish source, although in most cases allergies are caused by proteins in shellfish , and not in chitin, a carbohydrate from which glucosamine is extracted. The source of glucosamine may not be printed on the label, so it is advisable to contact the manufacturer.

Taking glucosamine with food may help reduce the ocurrance of digestive issues associated with glucosamine.

Other factors to consider

- Children, pregnant women and women who could become pregnant, should not take these supplements. They have not been studied long enough to determine their effects
- Glucosamine is an amino sugar, therefore people with diabetes should consult their doctor in advance.

What do past studies say about glucosamine?

Past studies show that glucosamine sulfate aids in the reduction of joint damage, and in regeneration of destroyed or degenerated joints.

Does glucosamine affect sugar levels?

“Even though glucosamine is technically a type of sugar, it doesn’t appear to affect blood sugar levels or insulin sensitivity. Studies refute the idea that glucosamine might worsen insulin resistence, therefore causing an increase in blood sugar in people with type 2 diabetes”.

Answer from Brent A. Bauer M.D. (Mayo Clinic).

Chondroitin

Chondroitin sulphate (C.S.) is part of a large protein molecule called ‘proteoglycan’ (see above under Glucosamine) which gives cartilage elasticity.

How is chondroitin sulphate manufactured?

It is usually manufactured from animal sources, such as shark and cow cartilage.

How does it work in our body?

Chondroitin stimulates joint function and helps with osteoarthritis.

Are there any side effects?

There are a few side effects to be aware of and these are:

- mild stomach pain and nausea, which are the most common ones
- also less common, constipation, hair loss, irregular heart beats and swelling of the eyelids or legs.

Is there anything else I need to be cautious about?

Consult your doctor, if you decide to take C.S. in addition to a blood thinning medication or daily aspirin therapy.

Homeopathy

Homeopathy (or homeopathic medication) is a medical philosophy and practice based on the idea that the body has the ability to heal itself.

Homeopathy was founded in the late 1700s in Germany by Samuel Hahnemann.

"Homeopathy is not a plausible system of treatment, as its dogmas about how drugs, illness, the human body, liquids and solutions operate are contradicted by a wide range of discoveries across biology, psychology, physics and chemistry made in the two centuries since its invention." (wikipedia.org).

Homeopathy's ineffectiveness has been backed by assessments done by reputable organisations such as the Australian National Health & Medical Research Council, the United Kingdom's House of Commons Science & Technology Committee and the Swiss Federal Health Office.

*On the other hand there are studies which prove otherwise, such as Rachel Roberts - a homeopath - who says "I know homeopathy works, not only because I have seen it with my own eyes countless times, but because scientific reasearch confirms it"

"By the end of 2008, 142 'randomised control trials' (the Gold Standard of medical reasearch) comparing homeopathy with placebo or conventional treatment, had been published in peer-reviewed journals. Seventy four of the studies were able to draw firm conclusions: sixty three studies had positive outcomes for homeopathy, while eleven had negative outcomes. It is usual to get mixed results when looking at a wide range of research results on one subject."

Valerie Lorentz-Poinsot, Director General of Boiron in France said, "We have conducted a large pharmaco-epidemiological study from 2006 onwards, which shows how much homeopathic medicine is in the public health interest." Those behind the campaign in France include world homeopathy manufacturer and advocate Boiron, and a homeopathy teaching authority CEDH (L'Ecoled'Ensignement de l'Homeopathie).

Personal experience – As I have limited personal experience of homeopathy I cannot vouch for either of these viewpoints.

Herbal Medicine

Herbal medicine is the use of plants for medicinal purposes. Plants have been used for medical treatments almost for ever, and it is still widely used today in many different parts of the world. H.M. includes fungal and bee products as well as minerals and shells.

The NHS gives a warning that "...just like conventional medicines, herbal medicines will have an effect on the body and can be potentially harmfull if not used correctly" So always consult you medical practitioner.

You should be aware of the following:
- they may cause problems if taken alongside other medicines
- you may experience a bad reaction or side effects
- not all herbal medicines are regulated
- evidence for the effectiveness of herbal medicines is generally very limited
- if you are pregnant or breastfeeding, consult your doctor first
- if you are due to have surgery, tell your doctor.

Personal experience - H.M can be very effective. The best example I can give is that of a very good friend of mine who had prostate cancer and went on remission for years after using a particular herbal medicine, cats claws. On the other hand though, some herbs like comfrey and ephedra can cause serious harm.

Note.- Farmacological medication is meticulously tested before they are licensed and can be made available. Homeopathic medicines and herbal medicines are not tested in the same way.

Always consult a doctor before taking any alternative medicines.

3. Mind and Body

a. Psychological Issues

Often depression, anxiety and stress come with back pain, especially chronic back pain. Researchers estimate that accompanying depression and anxiety occur in 20% to 50% of patients with chronic pain. While experiencing chronic pain, emotions and moods may be strongly influenced by the underlying physiology associated with the condition. It is likely that the doctor will ask if you have suffered from depression, anxiety, substance abuse or other problems currently and in the past.

b. Cognitive Behavioral Therapy

Cognitive Behavioural Therapy (CBT) is a type of psychotherapeutic treatment that helps patients undersatnd the thoughts and feelings that influence behaviour. CBT is commonly used to treat a wide range of disorders including phobias, addictions, depression and anxiety. It is a *talking therapy* that can help manage your problems by changing the way you think and behave.

CBT can help make sense of overwhelming problems by breaking them into five smaller parts, of which the main areas are:

- situations
- thoughts
- emotions
- physical sensationss
- actions

CBT is ...

- pragmatic – it helps to identify specific problems and how to solve them.
- very structured – you and your therapist discuss specific problems and set goals for you to achieve.
- Focusses on current problems – it is mainly concerned with how you think and act NOW rather than trying to tackle past issues.
- collaborative – your therapist and you will work together to find solutions to your current difficulties.

c. Mind Set – Positive Mental Attitude (PMA) - A Cognitive Strategy

Our thoughts can be positive or negative, strengthening or destructive, wise or reckless.

There are helpful and unhelpful ways of reacting to any situation, which are determined by how you think about them. For example, failing to pass an exam might lead to feeling a failure.

This could lead to feelings of depression and hopelessness, and as a consequence a decision to give up and not try again. You become negative, you allow negativity take over. On the other hand, taking a different attitude and saying to yourself, “I am not the only one, this happens to others too. I am not going to give up! I will try again!”

Positivity cultivates positive feelings such as love, compassion and goodwill towards others, impacting positively on emotional and physical health.

By cultivating a positive mental attitude (PMA) you can be in control of your mind set. A positive mental attitude is the belief that you can increase achievement and be in control of your thoughts, feelings, emotions and actions through optimistic or positive thought processes. If defeating and negative thoughts come to your mind, change them to helpful and positive thoughts.

Positive thinking is a discipline; the more you practice it and train your mind, the better you get at making positive mental statements and actions, which will lead to a sense of well being and optimism. Regular daily prayer and meditation (see Prayer and Meditation, on page 40) will improve mindfulness and positive thinking. It will also improve your health and sense of purpose.

Different ways to feel positive:

- start the day with positive affirmation
- focus on the good things
- turn failure into lessons/challenges
- focus on the present and take note of ONE positive moment every day
- remember no one is perfect and move forward
- find people you like and trust
- be active: either mentally or physically, ie: read a book, go for a walk, exercises at home, do something creative like drawing, painting, etc.
- Be kind – to do a small act of kindness (daily, weekly...)
- Make yourself useful and helpful to others a friend, a charity...
- Surround yourself with good and positive-minded people

- Be proactive and take action in regard to your health, happiness and future
- Don't look sideways – live your own life and don't compare yourself with others
- Be grateful – be content with what you have and count your blessings; try to be specific like people or moments for which you are thankful. Write five things for which you are grateful at a specific time each day.
- Put your gratitude into practice – attitude can change your behaviour, and behaviour can change your attitude.

d. Acceptance of living with chronic pain

Attitude has everything to do with quality of life while dealing with chronic pain. It is important to be realistic and positive, and avoid being too hard on yourself. One way to define acceptance could be "experimenting events fully, just as they are and not as they ought to be" (book: Overcoming Chronic Pain – see Biliography). No need to judge events and consider them as negative or positive.

People who suffer from chronic pain have the option to accept their limitations, without allowing the situation to define who they are. Being truthful and honest with yourself is important. Avoid doing what is now beyond you, while at the same time avoiding giving excuses for not doing something you could do by using creativity and lateral thinking. Challenge yourself to work out alternative approaches. ***Accept the things you cannot change, and focus on the things you can.***

Be realistic and recognise that your life situation is difficult but workable. View it positively and work out a helpful, practical and useful way to move forward. Acceptance will give you more confidence and control over your circumstances and your future. (see above under Mind and Body – Mind Set - PMA)

Personal experince - "Mens sana in corpore sano" (a healthy mind in a healthy body). This saying comes from satiric poems written by Roman author Juvenal, active in the first and second centuries. In those times, the meaning was to give great value and importance to the intelectual, physical and spiritual health/ fitness of an individual's well-being. To have a sound mind, body and soul is a very good goal in life.

I learnt through carrying constant pain over many years that both my mind and my attititude affect my physical wellbeing. I eventually learnt not to focus on my pain. My negative attitude affected my mood all the time. I was bordering depression many times. While researching my condition I learnt that as well as nerve tracts which carry pain signals upward to the brain there are also tracts coming down from the brain, which regulate the sensitivity of the spinal cord determining how much pain we perceive. I also noticed that my bad mood was affecting my chronic back pain, and making it worse. I made a conscious decision to control my moods by using Positive Mental Attitude (PMA) as a cognitive strategy and learnt to react to the situation I was confronted with, in this case my lower back pain and joint pains.

Having chronic back pain for so long (since 1961, and after my operation in 1989) I got to the point, around 1991-1992, when chronic pain forced me to accept that this pain would be lifelong presence in my life. I realised it was all about acceptance and started the process of changing my attitude by deciding to be truthful and honest with myself. I started the slow process of accepting my limitations and thought very carefully about what I needed to avoid, situations and activities I should not be doing, and most importantly, pacing myself (see Pacing below). I decided to focus on the things I could do rather than the things I couldn't. Finally, after I retired on medical grounds in the year 2000, I decided to take responsibility for my own condition by learning more about chronic back pain and how to manage it. I read a lot, I talked to lots of people, and was very eager to find out as much as possible.

I was determine to be resilient in the face of pain. I rejected the idea that I couldn't function well and not improve. I tried my hardest to push forward, mentally as well as phycically. I tried to engage with other people, look for opportunities to socialise and found that I became more confident as a result.

e. How to be more in control of your pain

In this section of Mind and Body we refer to the approaches that Psychophysiology offers and how they can be put into practice in order to be more in control of your pain. Psycho means mind and physio means body; how the mind affects the body and viceversa.

1.- Control of Breathing- Breathing is an unconscious action that you rarely think about, but over the years you may have developed poor breathing habits. Irregular breathing patterns, such as hyperventilation or overbreathing, can increase anxiety levels. When your body is calm, breathing is slow, regular and deep. But when anxiety levels are high, the opposite happens, breathing becomes fast, irregular and shallow creating feelings of panic. People who learn to breath calmly when they are feeling tense soon notice an improvement in their anxiety levels. The following guidelines will help correct overbreathing, and generally reduce tension.

- As soon as anxiety levels begin to rise, quietly tell yourself to 'calm down'. This sends a positive message to the brain.
- Slow down all your movements, because rushing around increases agitation.
- Calm your breathing deliberately and keep an even rhythm with a slight pause between the in and out breaths.
- Practice calm breathing at different times during the day so that you are aware of taking control.

See Appendix 3 (page 149), for step by step breathing exercises.

2.- Relaxation – Relaxation can help to reduce pain. Muscle relaxation is one of the most common cognitive techniques for symptom management. When relaxing muscle tension is reduced because the mind can affect the body. Relaxation can also allow the mind to become less active and focus on other thoughts rather than pain, worries, or other negative thoughts. There are different relaxation techniques ranging from simple breathing patterns, imagery techniques, self hynosis (see below) to meditation, Tai Chi and Pilates.

There are two broad types of relaxation techniques: deep relaxation and whole body relaxation.

- Deep relaxation – Deep relaxation is an excellent way to restore energy and boost your spirits. It may take several sessions to get it right. Relax muscles and practice slow quiet breathing, which sends calming messages to the brain and turns off the false reaction to danger. When there are no threats the body rests and restores itself.
- Whole body relaxation – This is the most common form of relaxation and produces pleasant results quickly. The technique works better if you create the right conditions and allow suficient time (about 20 minutes). If you prefer to relax with a teacher ask your doctor or your Healthcare professional.

See Appendix 4 for relaxation exercises to use at home, go to "Listening Exercise" (page 152) and Appendix 5 "Imagination Exercise" (page 153).

3.- Meditation/Prayer - Meditation therapy (MT) can manage pain and reduce stress and is something anyone can do. Those with a faith might refer to it as prayer/reflexion. When the brain rhythms slow down the mind enters a state or relaxation and rest, the heart rate, metabolism and breathing rates also slow down, and blood pressure lowers.

Natural pain killers called endorphins (see Activating Endorphins on page 107) are released into your system when your mind is calm like this. Recent studies have proven that M.T. is a very powerful way to help relieve pain without the many side effects that are found in some narcotics and other pain relieving drugs. Using M.T. to aleviate pain teaches the body to relax and focus on things other than the present pain, though it takes practice to become effective.

Pain can lead to anxiety and elevated blood pressure. Meditation helps reduce anxiety levels and bring down blood pressure. M.T. can help control pain, but can also improve health, and mental/emotional well-being. (see more under "Coping Strategies" on page 45)

Things to consider to help set up a good home environment.

a.- Creating a peaceful atmosphere – Create a quiet and peaceful space by putting your phone on silence and turn down the lights.
b.- Prepare and set up props – Although not essential cushions, or an easy chair may help you to feel comfortable.
c.- Water sound and candles – You may consider a small running water feature, a fountain, or a recording to listen to the soothing sounds of running water.
d.- Try to eliminate noise and distractions – Noise or loud music from neighbours, noisy traffic or workers outside can be very distracting. Use ear plugs if necessary.
e.- Play some calming music – Studies have shwon that playing music promotes relaxation. Sounds of nature or smooth classical music are very calming and great choices. Music can set the mood for reflection and contemplation.
f.- Have a comfortable temperature in your meditation/prayer-reflexion room by setting your thermostat where is most comfortable for you.

g.- Cleaning up your space is vital to creating a clean and calming atmosphere, by trying to minimise clutter in the room.

4.- Pacing is a valuable self help skill for managing chronic pain. It is simply a well thought out schedule to help you plan and monitor your daily activities. Pacing will help you do more over time, have more control over the pain, and have fewer set backs.

When you are having a good day doing too much might be counterproductive. On the other hand, when you are having a bad day, doing too little, spending most of the time resting, sitting or lying down, it is not very helpful either and may add to your pain. Over a long period of time of repeated inactivity muscles and connective tissue will become weak. Therefore, it is crucial to find a balance.

Personal experience – In the early 70s a friend, who knew about my chronic back pain, taught me how to slow down my breathing to help me physically and mentally. I find this really helpful, particularly at night, to induce sleep, as well as at other times.

Body relaxation is also good to quiet the mind, I learnt a particular technique after I retired in the year 2000 which you can refer to in the Appendix 3 (page 73). I did this regularly for quite some time as I found it very effective to relax my body and help me to have a good night's sleep, which I hadn't had for a long time. I wished I'd known this common cognitive technique earlier.

In 2002 my GP referred me to a physio, who gave me the exercises that I continue to do daily; he also recommended Taichi classes.

I attended Taichi regularly as I found some of the moves were very helpful.

I practiced guided meditation between 1970 and 1972, which was recommended by my doctor in Lima before coming to England.

I learnt about pacing myself in 2001. There are lots of different ways of putting this into practice (see below). It has been extremely useful in terms of managing my daily plan and helping me not to feel guilty or that I am a failure for slowing down or not finishing a task in one go. I had to change my mental attitude and accept the advantages of pacing myself which results in doing more over time, having more control over the pains, and fewer setbacks.

Some recommended pacing ideas:
- Focus on the things you can do, even if you are going to take your time, rather than the things you can't do at all. This will help you to avoid stress and frustration.
- Don't overdo it or push yourself, if you think you are having a good day, and risk a setback later.
- Avoid resting too much and try to move a little, as joints get stiff due to inactivity and possibly pain could set in.
- When resting your body keep your mind busy by reading, doing a puzzle, or anything that will keep your mind occupied and distracted from focusing on the pain.
- When you can't do what you want or ought to do, say to yourself, "This is only temporary, I'll be doing it tomorrow when I have rested". So look ahead, look forward to doing it! Be flexible and

understanding of your limitations to avoid feeling demoralised or frustrated. Be positive so you can build up your confidence.

- Make a realistic daily or weekly plan of activities. Prioritise according to what is important to you. Plan how you can easily achieve each of your goals, and how long you will spend on each activity. See example below.
- When doing a particular activity such as gardening, ironing or washing your car, see how long you can do it for before pain starts. Give yourself 5 minutes on a task, to start with that would be your quota. Then every time you do that same activity stick to your set timing for 4 to 6 weeks, then increase it a little say to 7 or 8 minutes; after a further 4 to 6 weeks increase it to 10, and so on.
- Monitor your plan and assess the advantages and disadvantages. If necessary readjust the plan.
- Focus positively on the fact that you are doing a given task, even if you cannot finish it in one go. Take as many rests as necessary, keep going, listen to your body and try to complete the task. The resulting success will give you more confidence and certainly great satisfaction.

5.- Resting - **Personal experience - As I have suffered from chronic back pain for 52 years, since my sports injury in 1961, and started having arthritis in 2002, I know how important <u>rest</u> is. We all need to plan to rest; rest allows time for the body to recover. I repeat that it is important to plan distraction strategies to engage the mind while resting in order to avoid thinking and focussing on aches and pains. I use a daily plan of activities including rest times distractions such as reading, writing letters or listening** to music. Initially I occupied my mind by undertaking a long term project: creating a board game. I included slots of time to do this as part as my overall plan of activities. In 2013 I decided to start doing reaserch to find out as much as possible about chronic back pain and arthritis. I started to monitor and record my condition in regard to pain, reaction and outcomes to various strategies in order to chart my progress or setbacks. This book is the outcome of this project.

I was a professional part time musician playing in a South American band called Caliche. We were together for 24 years and travelled all over the UK, both performing and doing music workshops in schools. Learning to play new instruments, which means I can now play ten different ones, was a distraction which brought me much joy, and led to aquiring useful new skills. I was able to continue composing music and songs, as I had done for my band for many years, after I had to retire from my main job as a Primary School teacher; a very effective distraction for a musician!

This Distraction Technique is not a treatment but a strategy which helped me a lot, and still does today (see "Stress Reduction Strategies" on page 89)

While I was working and suffering of back pain, I used to think that resting was a complete waste of time... there were so many things I wanted to do. Eventually I realised that resting is essential for healing.

After my operation in 1989 in Coventry I was very focussed and determined to implement various treatments and ways to improve my condition and physical and mental well being, I concluded that I had to include resting times as a very important part of my overall plan.

Ways for sheduling rest. - There are a few things to consider:

1. Decide which days or part of each day (morning, afternoon or evening) you are going to rest; whichever suits you best.
2. Draw up a plan of activities to suit you. Most importantly you need to decide how often you need a rest according to your condition. This plan should include all activities: commitments, leisure activities, social activities, and treatments or exercise either with a health professional or by yourself. Remember exercise is a vital component of the plan.
3. Be flexible and considerate with yourself in regard to being active and resting. If you need to reschedule your plan, do it. Only you will eventually know the right balance between activity and rest. Getting the balance right is what it's all about.
4. Do not allow the workload to be greater that your recovery. There are three things to consider: a.- physical activity (physical load), b.- stress (mental load) and c.- sleep at night, and rest breaks in daytime.

A good night's sleep and rests at intervals throughout the day are essential for recovery and healing.

There is a very common concern that too much rest due to the fear will lead to getting critically out of shape. I believe we need to be concerned about healing first. Regular resting does not mean stopping all physical activities and exercise as part of the overall plan. Remember exercise guided by professionals improves health proportionally to regular commitment.

There is the need of more research to be done in terms of how much activity and exercise is more effective, and also what strategies/tactics work best for fit people as well as for people with chronic medical conditions such as for example chronic back pain and arthritis.

Some concepts and ideas came from www.painscience.com

6.- Posture – The Alexander Technique Posture is extremely important. It was very useful to me at one time.

Personal experience - In 1980 I decided to look around for alternative ways to improve my chronic back pain condition. Recaping on what happened two years before, I tried various treatments with not much success. At St. Thomas Hospital (London), I tried two different treatments: three epidural injections and traction treatment. Both resulted in little relief which didn't last long, and I later found out that studies showed no evidence that either of these treatments were beneficial to patients. I was then recommended to try a 6 session course of acupuncture. After the fourth session I reported no improvement and the accupuncturist said there was no point in continuing.

In desperation I decided to try the Alexander Technique (this was in 1981) as recommended by a friend. After 5 sessions I concluded this was not a cure, but an educational process that

would help me manage my pain by avoiding bad postures and bad habits in moving my body.

The Alexander Technique (AT) is an educational process, teaching posture and movement, created by F.M. Alexander, to retrain habitual patterns. The main principles of the A.T. are "how you move, sit and stand affects how well you function"(www.nhs.uk). "The relationship of the head, neck and spine is fundamental to your ability to function optimally" (e.wikipedia.org).

Although I knew this wasn't a cure for my chronic back pain, I thought it might help me to avoid pain to some degree. What I learnt then, such as moving in a more balanced way, aligning my body when exercising, and avoiding bad postures that can aggravate my condition has become a habit from which I continue to benefit.

4. General Health Recommendations

a. What your body needs

Your body needs...
- energy
- nutrients, such as vitamins and minerals
- exercise – fitness
- good circulation and a stable blood pressure
- decontamination from: smoking, drugs, infections and so on.
- A good night's sleep and rest at other times.

Your mind needs:

- positive stimulation
- to be active (work, hobbies, leisure, etc.)
- to be positive – Positive Mental Attitude (PMA). The power of your mind can eliminate procastination and laziness and replace it with determination and perseverance.
- social interaction
- to feel useful to others
- to be stress free
- to generally enjoy life
- to have 'me' times
- to feel fulfilled by accomplishing targets and goals
- To have peace of mind by eliminating worry, hate and fear.

Worry creates anxiety which can lead to depression. Hatred creates bitterness and resentment which can lead to being ostrocised, feeling unloved and worthless. Finally fear creates negative attitude and introversion, which can lead to isolation and loneliness.

b. Stress Reduction Strategies & How to Help You Manage Stress.-

The following are just a few ideas. Most of these relaxation techniques/ ideas don't cost anything and are easy to put into practice. They will help because the mind can affect the body, while the body can affect the mind.

Living with chronic pain can be very daunting, sometimes to the point of not being able to cope, and possibly leading to more serious emotional problems such as despair and depression. We can lessen the intensity of our physical symptoms, including our emotions by using various distraction ways, some call them distraction techniques, an easy strategy to use.

What is the Distraction Technique? As the name implies, it is about distracting yourself, refocussing your attention (your mind) away from your symptoms by choosing not to dwell on them. Concentrating on a particular activity you are doing leaves less space in your brain to feel symptoms. Your brain can only focus its attention in just a few areas at one time. Pain sensations compete for attention with other things going on around you, so both physical and mental activity can distract your mind. When you commit your time to an activity, hobby or job that interests you, you are in control, you decide what occupies your mind. Keeping yourself interested and committed to do something you really enjoy is probably one of the best skills to be able to manage your condition better.

Coping Strategies

Everybody is different, we all have different interets, different ways to deal with difficult situations, and different ways of relaxing. You need to find out what strategies suit you. Some other natural pain relievering suggestions are:

1. **Meditation or prayer-reflexion** – Religious and spiritual beliefs are very important to many people; they can bring a sense of meaning and purpose to their lives. They will bring comfort in difficult times. Recent medical and scientific research suggests that people holding religious and spiritual beliefs may improve

their health and live longer, because both meditation and prayer help increase emotional well-being. When doing an overall weekly plan of activities, it would be helpful to timetable a time slot for prayer or meditation.

Just one simple example is to sit or lie down comfortably and close your eyes. Say something positive, preferably out loud, such as "I feel relaxed", and keep repeating it slowly. Push away any distracting thoughts and focus on those words of feeling relaxed.

If you are a christian, you could ask God to give you peace of mind and to relax your body, and keep repeating this; to help you to stay focus.

2. **Breathing exercises –** Find a comfortable position, when you are ready take two deep breaths, slowly inhale through your nose and exhale through your mouth, and concentrating on your breathing all the time.

   Now try this simple breathing exercise: Step 1- Inhale slowly through your nose to a count of 5; Step 2- Hold your breath for a count of 5; Step 3 – Exhale slowly through your mouth to a count of 5. Repeat this sequence a few more times.

3. **Slowing down –** By slowing down your thoughts, slowing down your behaviour and slowing down your activities, you will feel more in touch with all your senses, even taste if you have something to eat while you relax. The important thing is to focus on your senses.

4. **Connect with people** – Have a social encounter like talking to a close friend, or a relative, either face to face or by phone. Your mind will travel and go away from worries and negative thoughts. Feel the connection with that person and do not let any distractions get in the way. Talking things through with someone you trust will help you find solutions, particularly if they are supportive and understanding.

5. **Relaxing your body** – Concentrate and focus on relaxing each part of your body in turn, starting from your toes, then feet, calf muscles, knees and finish in your head. When you get to your face focus on eah part of your face including your jaws. When you focus on each part of your body, move that part a little and then relax it. When you get to the end, say to yourself "I feel totally relaxed". You may find you are so relaxed you fall asleep during the process!

6. **Laughter** – A good laugh lowers your body's stress hormones and releases brain chemicals called 'endorphins' (see later more on page 119). Talk to someone who will make you laugh or smile, read a funny book or watch a comedy.

7. **Exercise** – Exercise also lowers stress hormones. Try going for a walk; doing physio exercises at home, learning yoga, pilates or taichi. People who exercise regularly are less likely to experience anxiety and stress than those who do not exercise. Exercise is also known to boost confidence.

8. **Focus and remember things that were good for you in the past.** Then focus on those things (even if there are very few) that are very good now. If you are a Christian or a Muslim, tell Jesus/God how grateful you are for all those blessings you have received from Him, for all those opportunities you have had and for His love to you. Appreciate what you have, rather than what you don't have.

9. **Taking control -** Be in control and say to yourself "I can do this; I am in control; I will overcome this" Say it several times, be optimistic, be positive. Concentrate on the things you can control rather than on things you can't, and accept there are things you can't change.

10. **"Me Time"-** This is really important. Give yourself your own special time and treat yourself. Do things you really enjoy. It could be listening to music, socialising, relaxing, or going out with friends who make you feel relaxed and special. *Me time activities* will benefit your health rather than a self indulgence, so do not feel guilty about it.

11. **Go for a challenge -** For example learning a new language, learning to play an instrument; any new skill drawing, painting, woodwork and other crafts will build your confidence and will help you to avoid focussing on your aches and pains.

12. **Helping others –** There are various options: volunteering for a local charity, or for local campaign or support groups in your community. It could even be helping a neighbour or a friend in

need of help or support. Helping others is very rewarding and will give you a sense of achievement and satisfaction, especially if you make the person you are helping feel good.

13. **Release your inner endorphins -** They work by binding to the opioid receptors in your brain to block the perception of pain. See more: "Activating Endorphins" (pg. 107)

14. **Heat and Cold Treatment –** You need to know when to use heat and when to use cold. (See more: on pages 105).

15. **Other ideas –** I am sure that you will have your own ideas but these are some:

- Lighting a candle
- Listening to the running of water ie a fountain or a small water feature
- Changing your attitude – not letting little things annoy you and be philosophical about situations. We have made reference before about Positive Mental Attitude (PMA) – on page 74.
- Soaking in warm water.
- Enjoying the outdoors -10 to 15 minutes daily exposure to the sun helps the body produce vitamin D.
- Hugging, kissing, cuddling and making love will give you a sense of well-being and help you reduce stress and causing your body to release endorphins and relax.
- Getting enough sleep is critical to managing pain, stress, promoting healing and general well-being.

Personal experience – Apart from actions and coping strategies, events or circumstances in your life might help reduce stress. In my case one such event was meeting Ingrid in 1996 and getting married in 1999, my stress levels reduced massively as a result.

Another contributing factor to reducing my stress levels was that Ingrid was a Christian, which I could see helped her in all sorts of circumstances. After some exploration I also became a Christian and started to rely on God, which has also helped me cope with stress.

c. Stress may lead to depression –
Stress keeps you alert, motivated and gets you ready to respond to difficult situations; it helps your body to respond in a positive way and can improve your performance. Yet too much stress or chronic stress, can lead to depression.

The word "chronic" is used in medicine to refer to any disease or condition that persists over time or is frequently recurring. The term "chronic" is often used in contrast to the word "acute" which refers to a disease/condition that comes on rapidly.

Depression is common in people who have a chronic illness/condition. It is estimated that up to one third of individuals with a serious medical condition have symptoms of depression; they will inevitably have to adapt or change their lifestyles and daily routine, and could lead to stressful situations resulting in great sadness and despair. Depression caused by chronic illness can aggravate the illness causing a vicious cycle to develop. Depression is especially likely to occur when the illness/condition causes pain, disability or social isolation. Depression in turn can intensify pain, fatigue and the self doubt that can lead the patient to avoid social interaction. This is why socialising and connecting with people is so important. Individuals in this situation need to maintain contact with family and friends, enjoying one another's company, sharing activities, or learning something new together.

Personal experience - When suffering from a chronic and painful condition you not only have a physical battle to win but also a mental one. The mental battle is a great challenge requiring determination and strength to face alongside the physical challenges. Both must be tackled symultaneously in order to "win the war". Initially I didn't grasp this, but once I realised the importance of both I made great progress. After all this time I find I only need to use some of the strategies in situations when I find I am getting anxious or worried about a long term on going circumstance which is getting me down. I worked out I needed to be alert to 3 things I needed to eliminate from my mind: worry, hate and fear.

1.- Worry creates anxiety which can lead to depression.

2.- Hatred creates bitterness and resentment which can lead to being ostrocised, feeling unloved and worthless.

3.- Fear creates negative attitude and introversion, which can lead to isolation and loneliness.

By using the above mentioned strategies, such as meditation, prayer, reflexion, breathing exercises, connecting with people, relaxation exercises, hepling others and so on I have overcome much over the years; always remaining aware that mind and body have differing requirements.

d. My continually growing BIG PLAN -

Suggestions and Ideas of Things You Can Do At Home

Healthy Living – There are many things you can do to maintain a healthy lifestyle.

The body and the mind coexist in a to and fro relationship, one cannot exist without the other. With that in mind there are five things to consider:

1.- Keep physically active – We have already touched on this subject of movement being good for your body, and this includes informal activities such as walking as well as formal activities such as exercises (check with your physio or Health Professional).

Healthy body > Healthy mind.

2.- Keep mentally active – There are various things you can do such as: learning to play an instrument; learning a new language; learning a new skill ie crotchet, knitting, weaving, woodwork, painting, drawing and so on; going to museums; puzzles like crosswords or sudoku; fall in love with literature; listening to music; or socialise and connect with people (see above).

Healthy mind > Healthy body

3.- Healthy eating – We shall cover this next, see below.

4.- Avoid stress – more on this see: "Stress Reduction Strategies" (pg 44 above).

5.- Health Check ups – Here are some good reasons why regular check ups are advisable, especially if you have a chronic medical condition.

- To detect issues early, before a disease/condition gets worse.
- To keep your doctor and yourself up to date with your medical condition and general health. It also gives your doctor the opportunity to give you advice on how you can maintain/improve your health.
- To have blood tests in order to eliminate risks of several chronic diseases, these include cholesterol, diabetes, cancer, high blood pressure, anemia, HIV/AIDS, coronorary artery diseases, as well as the functioning of various body organs such as liver, kidneys, heart and thyroid.
- To help identify stress-related problems – Increase in stress and anxiety have been found to be directly related to a number of different problems/diseases, that are both physical and psychological. This is important for people with a chronic medical condition. Seek counselling and share your feelings; it may take courage to come out of your comfort zone, but it will be extremely beneficial.

For a reasonably healthy person check ups are a very good way of ensuring continued health, prevention is better than cure. But for people who have a chronic medical condition it is essential because they have to cope and learn how to manage and keep their condition under control as much as possible.

Health Check up list (www.healthcheckup.com)

- High blood pressure
- Body Mass Index (BMI)
- Breast and cervical cancer early detection
- Cholesterol cancer screening
- Oral health for adults
- Immunisations
- Skin cancer basic information
- Prostate cancer screening
- Viral hepatitis
- HIV/AIDS

Health check ups make you more aware of your health and gives you peace of mind.

Personal experience – I have always been into sports, mainly tennis, footbal, basketball and athletics. Three years after my back serious injury in 1961, I went back to playing basketball at national level. However by 1969 when I was 24 I could no longer carry on playing as it was extremely painful. Mentally it was very hard to accept retirement from sport at such an early age.

Maybe it wasn't a good idea to go back to play, I have been suffering constant pain because of the injury ever since.

At the time I just needed to concentrate on finishing my degree in architecture, which was another year and a half. I still thought I needed to keep active and living as normal a life as possible. My only possible sporting activity was leisurely swimming as even walking medium distances was becoming a problem.

Keeping my mind active has never been a problem for me as I have always had an inquisitive mind and read a lot. I continue to like acquiring knowledge about diverse things. I was interested in psychology and philosophy; qualified in architecture in 1969; photography, my favourite hobby; reading about famous people; learning about other cultures and travelling, and I embarked on science, my latest interest, in 2002.

At the age of forty (1985), I decided to try to eat healthily, keeping to foods low in sugar and low in fat because there was a worrying health history in my family. My dad suffered from palpitations nearly all his life; as have I since I was 18; he had high cholesterol levels, mild diabetes, and died of a stroke. My grandfather's medical history was very similar.

Following their footsteps, in 2010 (65 years old) I suffered a mini heart attack, and from then on have had to be even more careful. My heart condition was diagnosed as angina and AF (Atrial Fibrilation) also known as arrythmia, which I manage alongside my chronic back pain.

I have always tried really hard to avoid stress, though sometimes it is unavoidable, so have had to learn to manage it.

Healthy Eating – This is all about the nutritional value of what you eat and drink. There is a great amount of information about food and drink available in books, TV, the internet, and so on. We all know that eating nutritious food gives us energy and endurance, and it makes us feel better physically and emotionally. Healthy eating is about looking at the balance of the food you eat. These are basic principles to eat healthily in a balanced way:

- eat a wide variety of foods (see Food Groups – next page))
- eat regular meals – same time every day
- avoid snacking
- eat the same amount of food at each meal.

Eating a variety of food is important so that the body gets all the essential nutrients from the different food groups.

The nutrients we need are: proteins, carbohydrates, fat, vitamins and minerals.

The Food Groups

- Bread, potatoes, rice, pasta, and other carbohydrates. They provide a lot of the energy required for movement and warmth
- Fruit and vegetables – The NHS recommends to have five portions of fruit and vegetables each day. One portion is about a medium sized apple or banana, a bowl of salad or two table-spoonfuls of vegetables or pulses. These are a very good source of fibre.
- Dairy foods and alternatives – This group includes milk, cheese, and yoghurt. Butter is dairy but it is included in the 'fats' group. It would be healthier if you could choose reduced fat versions. You could still explore and try goat's and sheep's milk and cheese, as well as soya, oat or rice milk and cheese.
- Meat, fish, pulses, eggs and other proteins – This group includes the red meat beef, lamb and pork; the white meat such as chicken and turkey; and fish. There are alternatives to meat such as eggs, beans and pulses, and nuts – all these foods provide proteins. For

a healthier option chose lean beef. Be aware of the high levels of fat in sausages, pies, meatballs, fish fingers and fish cakes.

- Fats, oils and sugar – These foods very often are part of the ingredients for ready meals, take away meals, and packaged and processed food. Foods that could contain high levels of fat and oils are butter, margarine, spreads, cooking oils (extra virgin olive oil is a healthier option), mayonnaise and salad dressings. Foods containing a lot of sugar are biscuits, cakes, puddings, ice-cream, chocolates, sweets, crisps, sugar, and sugar sweetened drinks such as some juice and squash drinks, fizzy drinds such as coke, pepsi and others.

Most of us eat more than we need of this food group.

For more especific advice on best choices of essential oils that benefit people with arthritis. **Please go to Appendix 6 "Top 5 Essential Oils, especially for Arthritis" (page 154).**

- Fibre – Fibre is healthy and especifically good for your digestion.
- Water – We should all drink plenty of water. Studies have shown that drinking enough water decreases the body's inflammatory response. Inflammation is at the root of many medical conditions and diseases. The benefits of drinking water include: cells absorb nutrients dissolved in water; with fibre, it is essential for the proper progress of food and waste through your gut; it keep the kidneys functioning properly; it helps you to eat less; it maximises your energy; helps to control blood sugar; controls weight; among other benefits.

Please go to Appendix 7 "The Benefits of Drinking Pure Water" (page 156).

To summarise, here follows a General Guidance to Healthy Eating

- eating a variety of foods from all Food Groups
- eating at least 5 portions of fruit and vegetables (especially green) every day
- choose preferably food lower in fat – avoid or cut down frying and deep-fried foods e.g: fish and chips (from a take away) – they can be very high in salt. Too much sodium, can lead to a higher risk for developing high blood pressure.
- watching your cholesterol level
- watching high amounts of carbohydrates in a week
- reducing the amount of salt or sodium in your meals – avoid or cut down on salty snacks e.g: crisps, salted nuts; salty meat; stock cubes; some sauces high in salt like soy sauce.
- drinking water – Drinking plenty of pure water has lots of benefits. There are examples of people that have discovered that by drinking more water than they used to, their regular headaches stopped.
- watching your weight or BMI Body Mass Index – ask your Health professional.
- adding fibre gradually over a period of time
- eating more poultry – chicken, duck and turkey; eating less red meat – beef, lamb, venison and pork.
- avoiding or cutting down on sugar e.g: sweets, chocolate, cakes, biscuits, pastries, dried fruits, jam, marmalade, syrup, treacle and honey.

- Avoiding or cutting down on eating ready meals that are normally high in fat, sugar and salt. Many supermarkets now sell pre-prepared meals labelled as healthier options.
- Check food labels – food packages are required to provide nutritional information, which will help you to make healthier choices.
- Avoiding inflammatory foods, especially if you have a chronic medical condition such as arthritis.

Please go to Appendix 8, "Avoiding Inflammatory Foods". (page 158).

Please go to Appendix 9, "Foods to Avoid with Arthritis" (page 162).

Personal experience – After my mini heart attack in 2010, I decided to opt for better balanced meals. This included reviewing which foods I needed to add, increase, decrease or cut out. I found out that there are foods which I needed to avoid due to their inflammatory qualities, such as peanuts. Much later it was brought to my attention during one of my medical check ups that I wasn't drinking enough water, particular when the weather was mild or cold, which is most of the year.

All the information on healthy eating is something I have been learning slowly over the years; I intend to continue learning in the future.

Home Treatments – Here are some other ideas that might help you.

- The Heat and Cold Treatment

Heat treatment – It is normally used for chronic injuries or injuries that have no inflammation or swelling. Heat tends to make inflammation worse. If there is swelling or increased warmth in the painful area, you should not use heat. Considering that heat increases blood flow to the surface tissues, adding more heat may aggravate the situation.

Heat can be very helpful in relieving muscle spasm or tightness, helping you to become more flexible and relaxed. Heat will usually help if you feel cold, tense or anxious. Application: Apply heat for 15 to 20 minutes at a time, take a break of 40 minutes and then repeat again if necessary. If in a week there is no improvement contact your GP.

DO NOT use Heat Therapy – When the area is either bruised or swollen or both, it may be better to use cold. Heat should never be used in an area with open wound.

Cold treatment – The use of cold is currently recommended for acute soft tissue and joint and back conditions. Cold tends to "shut down" the blood supply temporarily close to the surface of the skin and therefore helps to decrease local inflammation or swelling that causes pain especially around a joint or a tendon. Basically what it does is numb the nerve endings in the painful area. Cold is particularly helpful for pain that is concentrated in one specific area that is sensitive to touch and/or appears swollen or warm. Cold may also help people with pain due to injuries, low back pain and joint pain.

If cold is not working for you, and you react to it by tensing up, you should stop the treatment immediately as it may aggravate pain symptoms. Cold therapy is also helpful in treating some overuse injuries such as repetitive strain injury, or chronic pain to reduce or prevent inflammation.

Application: Apply cold to the pain area for 15 to 20 minutes at a time, take a break for an hour then if necessary apply again. You can repeat the treatment again 3 or 4 times a day. If you do not get any relief with cold, wait a while and try heat; you may respond better to heat.

When not to use cold therapy – People with disorders that prevent them from feeling certain sensations should not use cold therapy at home because they may not be able to feel if damage is being done. This includes diabetes, which can result in nerve damage and lessened sensitivity. You should use cold therapy on stiff muscles or joints. You should not use cold therapy if you have poor circulation either.

- Recapping on the differences:

Acute pain is normally intense and short term, and could be as a result of a physical event such as a fall, a sprain or break. While chronic pain is long term and persisits for more than 6 months and does not respond to conventional treatments, such as arthritis, joint or back pain, and so on.

When heat therapy or cold therapy are used, caution must be taken to avoid burns and cold injuries.

Personal experience – I have been using both a heat bag and a cold pack for over 20 years and tend to use a tea towel between my skin and the bag/pack. This will allow you a few moments to adjust to the cold, and then you can remove the towel for the rest of the 20 minutes. After an hour the whole treatment can be repeated if pain persists. At times I still find it difficult to identify whether the pain I have needs heat or cold. Most times now I know, but it may take some "trial and error" to work out which therapy works best for your pain; this I have learnt from the experts. If not sure I use the cold pack first, if after 10 minutes there is no change, I use heat instead.

Activating Endorphins – Endorphins are natural pain killers, neuro-peptides and peptide hormones, found in your body produced by the central nervous system and the pituitary gland

See Appendix 10, "The Pituary Gland" (page 164).

These compounds once triggered will interact with receptors in your brain generating the feeling of pleasure in your body. What you feel is a tingling or goose bumps sensation that runs from the back of your head down your spine. In other words, endorphins produce a sense of well-being.

The word "endorphin" comes from endogenous, meaning "produced within the body", and morphine, a chemical substance derived from opium. Endorphins in turn, are neurotransmitters that are chemically similar to morphine. Some health professionals describe endorphins as being "endogenous opioid polypeptide compounds". In contrast with prescribed painkillers and other drugs, with endorphins there is no downside or side effects.

There are very many different chemicals in the brain known as neurotransmitters or endorphins. There are 4 such chemicals that work together to produce these sensation of bliss, happiness and well-being. These are: Dopamine, Serotonin, Oxytocin and Opiate Endorphins.

- **What is the effect of endorphins? -** The various benefits and positive effects include: lowering blood pressure; boosting the immune system; slowing down the ageing process; reducing pain; reducing anxiety and stress; it creates physical and emotional sensation of enjoyment and bliss; it enhances the pleasure of lovemaking; it enhances and improves your mood; it is relaxing for your mind and body; and it improves sleep.
- **How to naturally boost endorphins? - Triggers**
  Endorphin release generally happens when you: are injured; experience stress (either mentally or physically) or activate your natural reward system with activities such as exercise, love making, eating and drinking certain foods and drinks, and more, please see below. In addition to their analgesic, or pain relieving properties, endorphins are thought to be involved in controlling the body's response to stress, regulating contractions of the intestinal wall and determining mood.
- **Exercise –** The body produces endorphins in response to intense physical exercise. Many runners experience a state of euphoria while running. The release of endorphins varies from person to person but there is a common feeling associated with the term "runner's

high". Physical activity in general helps boost the production and release of endorphins in the brain.

- **Making love –** Making love (sex) is a very good way to release endorphins and feel good. According to the NHS sexual intercourse ("sexercise" as they call it), stimulates the immune system, can lower the risk of heart attacks, and help people live longer.

The most recent thinking is that exercise and love making can help treat depression (health providers often prescribe or advise exercise) and can reduce pain.

Please go to Appendix 11, "The Benefits of Making Love" - (page 165).

- **Food and Drinks -** There are certain foods and drinks that can help release endorphins. Everyone will have experienced certain foods and drinks which have a tendency to make you feel better because they contain nutrients that encourage the release of endorphins.

Low endorphin levels can be the result of certain vitamin and mineral deficiencies such as a lack of vitamin B, vitamin C and other minerals. If your body is not producing enough endorphins you might experience: depression; anxiety; moodiness; aches and pains; addiction (such as craving chocolate, alcohol or drugs in excess); crying over small issues and increased level of sorrow; incapable of accepting losses; extremely sensitive to pain; trouble sleeping or impulsive behaviour. So the opposite may be the case that the above mentioned symptoms may be reduced, alleviated and/or eliminated by endorphins.

Therefore eating a healthy diet is very important.

- eat enough protein to produce serotonin
- avoid processed food as they can interfere with brain chemistry.
- eat amino-rich foods: seeds, nuts, beans, lentils, peas, and sprouted grains
- eat green leafy vegetables such as broccoli, spinach, and kale.
- eat anti-oxidant-rich foods such as leafy greens, sweet potato, squash, citrus fruits, berries, alfalfa sprouts, broccoli.
- eat healthy fats – essential fatty acids in salmon, sardines, coconut, extra virgin olive oil, and avocado produce endorphin-promoting hormones.
- avoid excess alcohol and caffeine.

See Appendix 12, " Certain Foods That Help to Release Endorphins" - (page 166).

Personal Experience – I only found out about endorphins about 15 years ago (2005). There is much more readily available information on endorphins now than 15 years ago. I still remember the days when I woke up in the morning with pain and inflammation to my spine, and sometimes with added migrains, and had to get ready to go to work or for a concert with my band. I found out over time, that having a very hot shower was making me feel better, feeling a pleasurable sensation going down my spine as the warm water cascaded down my head and back, so when I had migrains I just stood under the shower for ages and I felt so much better afterwards.

Now I know that the pleasurable sensation I felt was due to the release of endorphins and other neurotransmitters.

Later on (2014), I found out that you can release endorphins at will by listening and/or performing music. In hindsight I thought "but I have felt these pleasurable sensations before while listening and performing music" (see below for more experiences).

- **Massage** – Research has shown that massage has a direct impact on lowering the levels of stress hormones and can boost "feel good" neurotransmitters like endorphins, dopamine, serotonin and oxytocin already mentioned. These 4 chemicals work in tandem and seem to be the stars of the show. They will boost your mood and give you a natural high feeling.

  Why does massage feel good? Most people who experience a good massage say it feels good. During a massage, tension and stress is released through the power of touch which will immediately cause a reaction in your brain releasing endorphins which will give you a natural high. As a result, stress hormones 'cortisol', (the stress related neurohormones produced by the adrenal gland) and adrenaline begin to decrease giving the overall effect of euphoria and bliss.

  The benefits are, diminished aches and pains, relaxed muscles and decreased inflammation. Massage helps improve circulation by moving blood more efficiently and releasing cell waste, like worn out proteins, faster than your body does naturally.

Personal experience – I experienced back and whole body massage only a few times after I retired, between 2002 and 2004. It was definitely effective, every time I went I felt relaxed and very good generally for a considerable length of time afterwards.

- **Music Therapy and Music be it Listening or Playing/ Performing –** Essentially, music therapy is the interaction between a therapist, a client (or clients) and the use of music. It has been proven to be effective with people of all ages and abilities. According to the Canadian Association for Music Therapy (M.T.), music therapy is the skillful use of music and musical elements by an accredited music therapist, to promote, maintain, and restore mental, physical, emotional and spiritual health. Music has non-verbal, creative, structural and emotional qualities. Professional Music Therapists can be found through General Practitioners, local Universities or by going on line. We will also comment on just listening or playing (performing) music, and how it can promote and help to improve well-being.

- **History –** The idea of music as a healing influence which could affect health and behaviour in a positive way is at least as old as the writings of Aristotle and Plato. Ancient civilisation artifacts as well as Biblical references suggest music was considered a powerful influence on physical health and well-being. (Gfeller, 2003). More recently, after World War 1, community musicians started to go to Veteran Hospitals around the country to play for the many veterans suffering both physical and emotional trauma from the war. The earliest known reference to Music Therapy appeared in 1789 in an article in the Columbiam Magazine. Benjamin Rush, a physician and psychiatrist, was a strong proponent of using music to treat medical diseases and conditions.

- **What are the effects of music?** – One of the best remedies for anxiety and stress is music, even known to reduce pain. It can be used to distract patients from unpleasant symptoms. It is widely recognised that music can create positive responses of joy and well-being and boost production of endorphins (see next section what studies show). Apart from listening and playing, studies show that music can make individuals feel a variety of emotions from happy and calm to energetic or relaxed.

- **What do studies say about Music Therapy?** – Various studies have shown that listening to music can be very beneficial and help to release endorphins, which creates the sense of feeling 'high' and relaxed. On the other hand high and lively music may create a sense of feeling joyful and confident. The type of music used can make different individuals respond in different ways, for instance relaxing music can alleviate anxiety and stresss levels quite efficiently.

  Other studies show that singing, dancing and drumming can also trigger endorphin release. The active performance of music generates the endorphin high as well. The findings of a University of Oxford study show that participatory music, such as drumming, triggers the release of endorphins, increasing the pain threshold. (www.x8drums.com/blog/drumming-and-endorphins).

See Appendix 13 "Drumming and Endorphins" - (page 170).

Sources on M.T. and Listening/Playing Music

- The Cochrane Library (a publication that reviews and reports on health care) looked at 14 studies involving 489 post op patients and their pain response to music. The studies found that while medication was the best form of pain reduction, music came in as second.
- Chiu & Kumar – 2003; Dunbar – 2008, 2009; McKinney et al – 1996 "A number of authors have suggested that the sense of elation that comes from engaging in music arises from the way music triggers the release of endorphins"
- Good *et al*, 2001
  "Music therapy can succesfully reduce post-operative-pain".
- Hilkiard, 2003
  "Music therapy can improve the quality of life in terminally ill cancer patients"
- Lusk & Lash, 2005
  "Research found that music alters specific physiologic responses, such as heart rate".
- Magill & Levreault, 1993
  "Music has also been found to alter mood and elicit relaxation responses".
- Stige, 2006
  "Music is able to elicit pleasure, which is assumed to motivate".
- Magill & Levreault,1993
  "Music as a distraction is able to alter thoughts, emotions or mood by inducing relaxation".
- Blood & Zatorre – 2001; Menon & Levitin – 2005.

"Neuroimaging suggests that the "thrill" or "chill" associated with music is due to the activity in the brain's reward centres. ...it is likely that involves endorphins, as well as the dopamines, commonly associated with the sense of thrill".

- S. Roberts – 2002 – Music Therapy for chronic pain.

  How music therapy positively affects perceived pain? There are several theories:

1) music serves as a distracter, 2) music may give the patient a sense of control, 3) music causes the body to release endorphins to counteract pain, and 4) slow music relaxes a person by slowing their breathing and heart beat.

- Weisenberg (1994) as cited in Megel, Houser & Gleaves (1998) suggested "distraction can be effective in moderating pain primarily through the cognitive component of the Gate-Control Theory of Pain (as mentioned above in Section: Chronic Pain – The Gate Control Theory of Pain, (page 13).
- McGill University, The Montreal Neurological Institute & Hospital (The Neuro), Quebec, Canada.

A study reported in Nature Neuroscience (January 2011) found that a chemical was released at moments of peak enjoyment. Researchers at the Neuro said it was the first time the chemical dopamine (mentioned earlier as one of the 4 'star chemicals'), has been tested in response to music. In this study dopamine levels were found to be up to 9% higher when volunteers were listening to music they enjoyed. For this study the researchers used PET (position-emission-tomography) and fMRI (functional magnetic resonance imaging) techniques to scan the brain of 8 participants (narrowed down from 217) as they listened to music over the course of three sessions. The result of the experiment was the release of dopamine (the feel-good chemical mentioned above). So when you experience an emotion while listening to music, your reward circuits are flooding your brain with dopamine designed to make you feel good and elated. This shows how researchers at the Neuro have been able to measure the release of dopamine in response to music that elicited "chills", changes in skin conductance, heart rate, breathing and temperature that were correlated with pleasurability ratings of the music.

"Chills" or "musical frissons" are a well established markers of peak emotional responses to a favourite piece of music; in simple words what some people feel when endorphins are released is a chill or shiver down the spine that starts at the back of your head.

The benefits of Music Therapy - It can help reduce pain, stress and anxiety, resulting in:

- Improved respiration
- Lower blood pressure
- Improved cardiac output
- Reduced heart rate
- Relaxed muscle tension.

According to Professor Suzane Hanser EdD, MT-BC, from Berklee College of Music, the music therapy protocol is designed to perform several functions:

- to direct attention away from pain or anxiety, distracting the listener with comforting music

- to provide a musical stimulus for rhythmic breathing
- to offer a rhythmic structure for systematic release of body tension
- to cue positive visual imagery
- to condition a deep relaxation response
- to change mood
- to focus on positive thoughts and feelings, and to celebrate life.

Please go to Appendix 14, "Musical Interventions in Music Therapy" - (page 172).

Personal experience – Listening, playing and performing music; which creates positive responses of joy and well-being; is something I have experienced throughout my life wihtout being aware there was a whole theory developing on this topic culminating in what is now known as Music Therapy.

As I have mentioned above I am a musician among other things. I started playing music at around 9 or 10 years old when I began learning to play the acoustic (or Spanish) guitar by watching two of my older brothers (we were 9 in total). Music has been part of me ever since. I first composed a piece of music when I entered a Music Competition for Composers in the late sixties, organised by channel 5 Panamericana Television, Lima, Peru. I continue composing to this day. I love all sorts of music: Peruvian Creolle music, Andean, jazz, classical music, folk music from many countries, rock and pop and so on. I have explained how some people can emotionally and physically respond to a favourite song or piece of music...well, I have felt those chills/shivers down my spine by listening to certain songs or pieces of music that

I absolutely love. It is such a pleasurable experience and now I know it's to do with endorphins. It really is so amazing!

* TENS Machine (transcutaneous electrical nerve stimulation) – Is a method of pain relief involving the use of a mild electrical current. The main purpose is to help reduce pain and muscle spasms caused by a range of conditions, such as arthritis, period pain, pelvic pain, knee pain, neck pain, back pain, sports injuries and other joint pains. Tens is **not** a cure for pain; it only provides a short term-relief while using the TENS machine, but it is very safe and worth trying in addition to other treatments.

  It is always a good idea to consult with your doctor; particularly those who may have other underlying health conditions; as they could refer you to a physiotherapist or pain clinic. It is highly recommended that a physiotherapist adjusts the settings correctly for you, according to your individual condition. The physio will also advise how and when to use it, and discuss whether TENS machines are available on loan. TENS machines are readily available and are not too expensive.

The benefits of a TENS machine are:

- **Pain relief –** The impulses aid in the release of endorphins that relieves pain naturally without any side effects
- Effective and efficient complementary therapy
- Portable and easy to use
- Increases circulation and healing
- Improves sleep patterns
- Benefits for spasms and knots

– Reduces inflammation
– Less fatigue and tiredness - stimulating muscles and nerves greatly reducing fatigue levels.

DO NOT USE TENS WITHOUT FIRST SEEKING MEDICAL ADVICE IF:
– you have a PACEMAKER or any other type of electrical or metal implant in your body
– you are pregnant or there is a chance you might be prgnant
– you have epilepsy or a heart problem.

* Laughter – Laughter is immensily therapeutic for body, mind and soul, with the added benefit of being free and joyful. Laughter is good for your overall health, especially because it boosts the immune system, improves circulation and releases endorphins. What's more, scientific studies show that laughter has positive effects on the heart, blood vessels, stress hormones, mental health and family relationships.

  Doctors have been looking at humour and laughter to **distract** from pain for centuries. Happy **distraction** can be a great contributor to pain management and pain reduction. Laughter is easily accessible. Distraction is one of the various easy to use cognitive strategies available. It is all about training your mind's attention away from your symptoms. Because our minds find it difficult to focus/concentrate on more than one thing at a time, we can train our minds to focus attention on something other than our bodies, thus diminishing the intensity of our physical symptoms.

When you laugh your levels of cortisol and adrenaline drop resulting in immediate reduction in sensitivity to pain. A hearty laugh contracts dozens of muscles, that tensing-relaxing sequence of action leads to a pronounced release.

See Appendix 15, "The Proggressive Muscle Relaxation", (page 174).

How laughter activates endorphins – Good strong laughter releases endorphins, the natural brain chemicals we have mentioned before. Because laughter changes your breathing pattern, you begin to draw out your exhalations, and this will exhaust your abdominal muscles, triggering the release of endorphins in the same way physical exercise does.

Social Laughter

Researches from the Turku PET (Position Emission Tomography) Centre, University of Turku, Finland; the University of Oxford and Aalto University, Finland, have revealed how social laughter leads to endorphin release in the brain. The pleasurable and calming effects of endorphin release might signal safety and promote feelings of togetherness, the establishment to social bonds. The study was conducted using PET scans (Position Emission Tomography). Participants were injected with a radioactive compound that adheres to opioid receptors in the brain. Using PET imaging the researchers were then able to monitor the release of endorphins and other peptides.

* Hot showers – Hot showers are good for relaxation. They can relieve tension and soothe stiff muscles. A hot shower works like a mini-

massage on your body – head, neck, shoulders and back. Studies have shown that taking a hot shower can boost your oxytocin* (see below) levels and ease tension and anxiety. A hot shower also acts as a natural decongestant to relieve colds and respiratory symptoms, since the hot steam moisturises nasal passages. Best of all a hot shower can actually relieve pain if you aim at certain parts of your body, namely back of the head, neck shoulders and especially the back of your ears. If you stand directly under the shower and let the water hit the top of your head, letting the water trickle down in all directions round your head, down your face, the sides (where the ears are), and back of your head, you will feel a pleasurable tingling sensation which is the sign of endorphins being released.

Warning for those who might have heart problems! Heart attacks happen very often in the shower. Always make sure the water temperature is bearable rather than too hot. The safest way is to start by wetting your feet first, then your legs, and gradually going up to your shoulders and finally your head, so the body aclimatises and there isn't a sudden rush of hot water on your head, which could lead to a stroke or heart attack.

Personal experience – I discovered these strategies of laughter and having hot showers in the mid-1990s and have been using them ever since. I have often gone into the shower in pain and came out feeling a lot better than I went in. I, like most people, have always liked the idea of having a good laugh. It makes you feel good and more relaxed. You can enjoy laughter even away from social situations, the most obvious being by watching a

comedy, comedian or movie, or reading a book that *you* find very funny.

When taking a hot shower, always ensure that it's a comfortable temperature to you individually, being sensible and do not overdo it, a hot shower can dry and irritate your skin, aggravate some skin conditions such as Eczema, and can cause itchiness and increase blood pressure.

* Oxytocin is a hormone that also acts as a neurotransmitter in the brain. It appears to be connected to human emotions and the regulation of child birth and breastfeeding. Oxytocin is thought to be released during hugging, touching and orgasm in both genders. Greater amounts of oxytocin hormone levels appear to be associated with greater relaxation. It also appears to help reduce stress response and reduces anxiety in people who suffer from it.

Dopamine, Serotonin, endorphins and oxytocin are all "happy" neurotransmitters in the brain that we have mentioned before.

– **Other Creative/Alternative Solutions** which are easy to put into practice.

- Good mattres/Good sleep – It is well known that being healthy is a matter of keeping a healthy weight, eating healthy foods and doing the right exercises for your body. Although they are important, there are other factors, such as a good night's sleep, that will improve your overall well being. I personally consider a good night's sleep among the top five most important factors alongside keeping your mind/soul healthy, and the three above mentioned.

A good sleep gives your body a chance to relax physically and mentally, as well as repair itself. The quality of sleep can be improved with a good mattress. A quality mattress could be a good investment towards your well being. Selecting a mattress is very personal, Dr. Decker PhD, professor at Georgia State University, and spokeman for the American Academy of Sleep Medicine, recommends one that is neither too firm nor too soft.

Aim for about 8 hours of quality sleep each night. If you are having trouble sleeping at night, some of the relaxation exercises recommended in this book might help (see pages 152 and 153). Lack of sleep could be detrimental for your well being, make it harder to concentrate on tasks, can cause mood changes, and could even make you more accident prone.

Last but not least a good quality pillow is also essential for quality sleep. As with a mattress this is a matter of personal choice, though one that is neither too hard nor too soft is recommended.

Personal experience - After retiring on medical grounds in the year 2000, I was recommended to use a back support belt, which I did at all times. I had not yet started doing exercises and was still complaining to my doctor about back pain and was taking pain killers as a result. A doctor friend suggested I ask my doctor to refer me to a physio who could teach me the right exercises for my condition. I had been recommended exercises in the past but

I did not take them seriously, maybe because I didn't believe that they would be beneficial. Using the support belt all the time and not doing exercises, resulted in my muscles, nerves and ligaments becoming lazy and weak. I started doing my exercises as directed by my physiotherapist every day. I learnt exercises that were going to strengthen both my back muscles and my abdominal muscles. After a few months I stopped using the suppport belt. It took a long while before I felt the benefits of doing exercises, but my perseverance was rewarded. I continue doing the exercises and don't think I would ever stop as I fully understand it is the only way to remain mobile and active.

If you are recommended by a physician or other health professional to use a support belt or brace on any of your joints, do not use them all the time and be sure to regularly follow the exercise regime set by your physiotherapist.

The market is full of back supports and joint braces, so you won't have a problem in getting what you need. You could ask your physio for advice in this regard.

- Protecting your heels, sciatic nerves and back – One very common nerve irritation is sciatica. When you have sciatica, the sciatic nerve, which runs from your lower back, across your buttocks, and down each leg, can become irritated and cause symptoms such as a pins and needles sensation, stinging, numbness, burning, an electric shock or pain.

These symptoms can manifest as:
- pain in the lower back
- pain in the saddle area aggravated by sitting for too long
- burning or pins and needles sensation in the leg
- weakness or numbness in the leg or foot
- difficulty in moving the legs or feet
- shooting pains going along the back of your legs, sometimes described as an "electric pain".
- shooting pains coming from your heels up along the back of your legs causing difficulties in walking, sometimes referred as "sciatica heel pain". Your heel pain can be a result of problems with pressure on the L5 – S1 nerve root.

Pain can be caused by damage to the nerves and by many other causes, including:
- inflammation
- trauma
- chemicals
- compression of the nerves
- infections

Personal experience – In 2010 I started to look for insoles, specifically to protect and cushion my heels, because I was finding it more and more difficult to walk, even for short distances. The pain on my heels was very bad. I started using some gel cushion heel insoles which were very popular at the time, and they helped a little for a while. Then I decided to put two cushion heel insoles on each shoe, and it was even better. About two years later I found some better insoles, which were expensive but worth it.

They are easily accessible on line from podiatry and chiropody websites, or from a footcare specialist shop. These expensive cushion heel insoles are absolutely brilliant. I am now able to go for longer walks than before.

* Keep searching - Learning new skills and finding new solutions can take time. Taking control of your chronic pain might take a long time. Practice and perseverence are as essential as trying different skills and possible solutions. This can be done systematically through action planning and monitoring results to see what works for you. The more you learn about your condition the easier it will be for you to manage it.

5. Other Therapies & Health Professionals

Chiropractic - is a non-conventional treatment sometimes considered complementary or alternative medicine, although some would say it now qualifies as mainstream. A chiropractor diagnoses and treats musculoskeletal disorders, using manipulation, to help relieve especifically bone, muscle, nerve and joint problems, which can affect other organs. They also advise patients on how to help themselves through exercises, ergonomics, general health and lifestyle.

Chiropractors are not necessarily physicians or doctors, but they are musculoskeletal specialists. Chiropractic is based on the principle that the body can heal itself when the skeletal system is properly aligned and the nervous system is functioning correctly.

If the bones of the spine are not articulating as they should, the nerve transmission is disrupted and causes back pain as well as pains in other areas. Chiropractic treatment carries none of the risks associated with surgical or pharmacological treatment. Chiropractors are excellent diagnosticians, and finding the cause of the symptoms is half the battle to resolving the problem.

Personal Experience – After my operation in 1989 I was able to go ahead with my PGCE course to become a primary school teacher as I had hoped and planned. As soon as I finished the course in June 1990, I got a job at Hearsall Community Primary School. I was still suffering from chronic pain at a more manageable level, but it was still a struggle.

In 1991 I was recommended to go to a chiropractic clinic and I also went to see a physiotherapist, who taught me exercises to do every day. With my busy life as a teacher (maybe this was an excuse) I didn't do my exercises very often and once again didn't take it seriously.

I heard that this particular chiropractor helped a previously wheelchair-bound patient to walk again, so I went very optimistically. On the first day there was no treatment, only an x-ray and an assesment. I had weekly appointments for about 2 months, and then once a month for a while. Once the chiropractor thought I was on track he told me to make an appointment whenever I needed it. I went on year after year, but I was going slowly down hill.

By the year 2000, I was in such a bad way that I had to retire on medical grounds. I was house bound, not being able to walk very far, for about a year. I went back to my chiropractor, and in about 9 to 10 months I was so much better that I decided I might be able to do some work and opted for a self-employed job working from home. I still continued seeing my chiropractor about once every 6 weeks or when I felt necessary. In 2002, I was referred to yet another physiotherapist, who explained clearly why I should follow my exercise routine to the letter. (for more on this go to Exercises section (page 58, 152, 153 and 172).

Osteopathy – is a type of physical therapy with the aim of detecting, treating and preventing health problems, by moving, stretching and massaging a patient's muscles, nerves and joints. According to the General Osteopathic Council (GOC), osteopathy "is based on the principle that the well-being of an individual depends on the skeleton, muscles, ligaments and connective tissues functioning together".

The osteopath's aims are:

- To increase the mobility of joints
- To relieve muscle tension
- To enhance the blood supply to tissues.
- To help the body heal itself relying on the body's healing mechanisms.

People seek osteopath treatment to get help with conditions such as:

- back pain
- neck, shoulder, elbow and other joint pains
- pain from arthritis

- pains related to the pelvis, hips or legs, from bad posture or work strain.
- Sports injuries

Manual therapy techniques are used by osteopaths as well as by physiotherapists and chiropractors. The osteopathic techniques are chosen on the individual patient according to the symptoms they have reported. Techniques include:

- massage – to release and relax muscles
- stretching stiff joints, nerves and ligaments
- articulation/manipulation – where your joints are moved through their natural range of motion
- high-velocity thrusts – short, sharp movements to the spine.

Osteopathy is a regulated health profession in the same way as medical doctors. Osteopthy is not widly available on the NHS (at the time of going to press). You can contact the General Osteopathic Council to enquire about osteopaths in your area.

Before going ahead, discuss it with your doctor.

Personal experience – My only experience with an osteopath was in 1998 when my chiropractor was on holiday and I needed help. A friend recommended him to me, but unfortunately the osteopath put my back out. The injury he caused was so bad that I was off work for 6 weeks as a result. I am not suggesting all osteopaths are ineffective, but each lower back chronic condition is unique, and I ended up worse through this experience. It took my chiropractor a few months to remedy the damage.

Acupuncture Is a traditional form of medicine that's been used succesfully for over 4,000 years in China and can bring your body back into balance naturally. This traditional chinese therapy is based on the idea of energies in the energy called 'qi' (pronounced 'chee) through the body's functional systems, such as the nervous, respiratory, circulatory, muscular and digestive systems. When the *qi* is blocked somewhere, pressure piles up in local tissues causing pain. If *qi* is not reading some part of the body, the fortification provided by the *qi* is reduced and disfunction in this area will produce pain. The acupuncturist selects the appropriate acupuncture points to promote the flow of *qi* in the channel to break the blockage.

Acupuncture can effectively manage headaches/migraines; muscular pain in neck, back and limbs; period pain; labour pain; cancer induced pain; pain caused by herpes (shingles); trigeminal neuralgia and sciatica.

Acupuncture stimulates certain body points, known as the acupuncture points, to induce the nervous system to release chemicals in the muscles, spinal cord and brain, including endorphins such as encephalin and other neurochemicals. These natural chemicals may either change the pain experience, or trigger the release of other chemicals and hormones that influence the body's own internal regulating system. Acupuncturists use pre-sterilised single-use disposable needles at various pressure points, to encourage the flow of chemicals and electrical information through the body. Chinese medicine states: "where there is free flow, there is no pain".

Acupuncture needles do not cause pain, harm or discomfort. The benefits are:

- It stimulates the nervous system by encouraging the free flow of chemicals and electrical information.
- It releases neurotransmitters endorphins and other chemicals to improve pain.
- It releases hormones that send messages regulating the on/off mechanisms of various nerve endings
- There are no side effects.
- It is a safe procedure in the hands of a qualified and registered acupuncturist and is painless.

Always consult you medical practitioner who can direct you to someone who is qualified and regulated (see next point below). Acupuncture should not be used on anyone suffering from a bleeding disorder or anyone using blood thinner medication such as aspirin or warfarin. Bear in mind that there are some people that may not respond to acupuncture. If you don't feel any improvement after 3 sessions, then it is not for you and you will be advised not to carry on with the treatment.

Acupuncture clinics and acupuncturists are regulated in the UK in a different way to other health professionals. Acupuncturists in the UK are not subject to statutory regulation although they need to join one of a number of organisations on a voluntary basis.

The following are the most well known and recognised organisations that offer membership to accupuncturists, subject to them attaining a certain level of qualification:

- The British Acupuncture Council (BAC)

- The Acupuncture Association of Chartered Physiotherapists (BRCP)
- The British Medical Acupuncture Society (BMAS)
- The British Academy of Western Medical Acupuncture (BAWMA)
- The Acupuncture Society.

The general public can also approach these organisations for information on registered acupuncturists near their area.

Personal Experience – I have had only a couple of experiences with acupuncturists. One was in 1974, when I was also trying traction and epidural injections at St. Thomas' Hospital in London. The acupuncturist I was referred to explained it was not worth continuing as there was no change after four sessions because some people do not respond to acupuncture. I was clearly one of them.

The second time, when I was living in Coventry in 2004, I had the same experience, which confirned what I had been told thirty years before.

Spiritual Healing Techniques – Prayer and meditation, the two more common methods, remain the oldest of self-management communication tools and are practised in many parts of the world. Religious and spiritual beliefs are essential for many people. Beliefs bring a sense of meaning and purpose to life. It can help put things into context and set priorities. It may help us find comfort in difficult times, or to feel more confident and positive, and can motivate us to make necessary changes.

Scientifically conducted trials in laboratory situations show that people experience relaxation responses when praying or meditating. Blood pressure, heart rate, and levels of stress hormones drop at the same time as brain waves associated with relaxation increase. These physiological changes reduce anxiety and increase blood protein levels in the body, indicating a healthier immune system. In addition, prayer and meditation also provide a form of distraction for people with long-term health conditions.

Definitions

Prayer is a communication process that allows someone to talk to God or another deity. For some, prayer is the practice of the presence of God; it is the moment when pride is abandoned, hope is lifted, supplication is made and gratefulness is forthcoming. It is a time of having an intimate conversation with God and sharing feelings, needs, desires, and concerns with God.

The act of prayer is of great significance for believers of all religions and faiths, whatever their inspiration, revealed or otherwise. Ludwig Feverbach, a 19th century German philosopher, summed it up: "The most intimate essence of religion is revealed by the most simple religious act: prayer". Meditation is the practice of turning your attention to a single point of reference. The word meditation comes from the Latin word 'meditari' which could mean three things: to reflect, to study, or to practice. There are many forms of meditation which can involve focussing on breathing, body sensations, on a particular word (ie. love, peace...) or phrase known as mantra. During meditation it is important to turn away from distracting thoughts and focus on positive thoughts in the moment, or focus attention on nature (ie. a flower, cascading water, a landscape...) or a particular object. Meditation is effortless and can lead to a state of 'thoughtless awareness'. Its main aim is to calm and silence the mind to achieve a stable emotional state. Studies show that meditating even for a short period of time, say 10 minutes, can increase the brain's alpha waves (associated with relaxation) and decrease anxiety and depression.

Some words closely associated to meditation are contemplation, thought, thinking, pondering, reflection, concentration.

What is the difference between prayer and meditation? - No matter which faith you belong to, the way to reach your inner self and attain peace with oneself and God (or other deity) is often through prayer and/or meditation. The way to achieve a balance of energy of body and mind, and peace of mind is through prayer and meditation. Although these two practices are very similar and overlap, there are subtle differences:

- Prayer is a method of speaking out our heart to the Divine, while in meditation you learn to medidate with your inner voice.
- There are two entities in prayer while there is only one in meditation.
- Praying is like having a conversation with God, while meditation is looking inwardly.
- Prayer is about listening for guidance and asking God for something while in meditation this does not happen.
- During prayer, the believer is like a child in front of his mother or father while in meditation is just sitting in the deity's company.
- In prayer you experience the presence of God (or other deity) and can have an intimate conversation with Him, while in meditation you don't.

- In meditation the goal is to attain a deep sense of relaxation , which is not the aim of prayer.
- Meditation is a pracrice when an individual tries to concentrate on their inner self, while in prayer you concentrate on your relationship with God (or other deity).

In short: prayers look up, meditations look in.

Other cognitive strategies – We have already mentioned above two of the various cognitive strategies available. One is Positive Mental Attitude (PMA) or positive thinking. Please go back to section, Mind Set – Positive Mental Attitude (page 74) to refresh your memory.

The other one is the Distraction Technique which is a strategy that directs your attention away from your symptoms. Please go back to the section, Stress Reduction Techniques... What is the Distraction Technique? (page 85-90).

There are two more cognitive strategies that could be under the category of spiritual strategies. These are:

- **Centring Prayer** – There are many kinds of prayer, but there is one form that might suit you and bring positive effects in your life.

Please go to Appendix 16, "Centring Prayer", (page 175) and it explains how to do it.

- **Mindfulness Meditation** – The main purpose of the different types of meditation is to quieten the mind, and it is a useful technique for people with long-term conditions such as pain, stress, tiredness and short of breathness.

Please go to Appendix 17, "Mindfulness Meditation", (page 177), and it will be explained.

- **The History of Prayer and Meditation** – The origin of both prayer and meditation is seen mainly in religious contexts throughout history. The act of prayer itself is of great comfort and significance to believers of all faiths.

For more information on the history, origin and development of these two practices.

Please go to Appendix 18 , "The Origins and History of Prayer and Meditation in our World" (page 179).

6. Summary of my story

Year	What happened
1945	I was born in November this year, in Lima, Perú. I was the 5th of nine children. I lived in a Catholic country, in a Catholic household (something relevant to be mentioned- see later on).
1961	I had my back injury playing basketball. I broke two vertebrae (L5 and S1). Two specialist Doctors from the

Mayo Clinic saw me and decided not to operate and recommended to go to see a physiotherapist.

1962 I finished school (Colegio Santa Maria)

1963 I went to see a family doctor who prescribed valium, a strong painkiller and anti-inflammatory medication. Valium was not recognised as an adictive drug at the time, and it was freely prescribed.

1964 I started to study Architecture (Facultad de Arquitectura – Universidad Nacional de Ingenieria – Lima). I was recruited to join Club Regatas Lima's basketball team. I started playing basketball again. This team was one of the top teams in Peru's top division.

1965-66 Two very tough years for me, studying architecture full time and playing basketball at a very high level. We won the championship in both years. The following year our two best players went to play basketball to the U.S.A. It was at the end of 1967 that I recognised I had become addicted to valium, and consulted my doctor for help to come off it. It took me about 7 months to 'kick the habit'.

1967-68 Another two very tough years. By the end of 1968 I had two things happening, one good and one bad. The good one was that I finished my studies in Architecture, and the bad one was due to my back pain I had to retire on medical advice from playing basketball or any other sport all together.

1970-73 After graduating as an Architect I started my first job working for the Ministry of Education of Perú designing schools for the whole country. I worked for nearly three years there. I won a scholarship from the British Council to study a postgraduate course on Designing & Planning Educational Buildings.

1973-75 While studying at UCL (University College London) I was still experiencing the same pains and other symptoms as previously, a bit more severe this time as it was compounded with stress. I was referred to St. Thomas' Hospital where they tried different procedures such as traction, epidural injections, medication and acupuncture. In October of 1975 I returned to Lima, Peru.

1975-77 These 18 months in Peru were very hard for me because I had to deal as best I could with my symptoms, and also because there was a lot of political unrest there at the time. So I returned to England in April 1977.

1977-84 I experienced a further 7 difficult years in London. I was referred to East London Hospital where a back specialist told me there was nothing he could do, but recommend to see a physio. I went for a couple of sessions, but didn't take the exercises seriously. A friend recommended me to go to a specislist in the Alexander technique which offered minimal help. Around 1980 I started playing in a South American band in London. At the end of 1984 I moved to Coventry with my young family.

1985-88 My condition started to deteriorate more and more. At the end of 1985 I met a Chilean who asked me if I wanted to join a South American band. Caliche, the band, was based in Birmingham. I joined Caliche that year and 12 months later we were travelling around the UK performing in concerts and running music workshops although my back was still playing up. I could hardly walk to the local shop 100 meters away from home at one point. By the end of 1988 I went to see a specialist at the hospital and he said the only thing he could offer was an operation. I agreed to have a fusion operation, although the success rate for this type of operation was only 35% at the time. The operation went reasonably well and I was a lot more mobile and active after a 6 months long rehabilitation period.

1989-90 At the end of that year, I started the PGCE (Postgraduate Certificate of Education) course at Warwick University, to become a primary school teacher, something I had always wanted to do.

1990-99 As soon as I graduated I was offered a teaching post at Hearsall Community Primary School, a local school in Coventry only a 15 minutes walk from home. In my first year I was doing quite well with my back condition most of the time. A friend recommended a chiropractor who helped me to get through my first year. I went to see him for a *body 'MOT'* mostly every couple of months, more often when I was in a bad way. 1996 was a fantastic year for me. I met Ingrid, the lady of my dreams, and got married in 1999. The following years went by and I was visiting my chiropractor 2 or 3 times a year. In '98 and '99 I was definitely going down hill and finding coping with my back issues very difficult. I was off work quite a lot as a result. I had reduced my teaching hours to part time and continued playing with my band and travelling quite widely, and all over the UK, Denmark, Spain, Portugal, Italy, Cyprus, Georgia, and so on.

1999 I was starting my 10th year as a teacher when in November I suffered a very serious incident, as I went to sit with the children at one of their small tables to give them some teaching support. Twenty minutes later I tried to get up and couldn't; I felt a horrific pain on my lower back and right leg. I was off work, hoping to return soon, but it was not to be.

2000-01 I had to retire in 2000 on medical grounds. As a result of my retirement our joint income plummeted though my wife was still working and we were struggling financially. I had my back issues to contend with as well. I asked my doctor to refer me to a physio once again, which is when I learnt about the very good exercises for my lower back mentioned in the text. This is the year when I decided I was going to diligently find out more about my chronic back condition, through books, the internet, and talking to specialists in this field. At the end of 2001, we decided to go for a self-employed job working from home. My wife was still working but helped with the business as much as she could. The process of learning all about my condition and how could best help myself started slowly mainly because I was busily working on the business which took up a lot of my time and energy.

2002-03 The deterioration of my condition continued and I was finding it quite difficult. After about a year after I started my daily exercises I noticed a great improvement and decided to add a few more different exercises to help my hand, knee and ankle joints (this is when my arthritis started). I did most of my exercises on the bed first thing in the morning which took about abour 45 minutes, as well as other exercises standing up. In 2003 I gave up prescribed medication. My physio also recommended Taichi, which I tried but found that some of the exercises were causing me discomfort and pain so I stopped going to Taichi but continued doing a few of the exercises I found helpful.

2006-07 By this time, I was clear of joint pains my arthrits was gone. In my view this was the result of many things I did, but the main ones were: the combination of taking oils (glucosamine sulphate and evening primrose oil mentioned above) for my back and joints, doing my exercises diligently, plus avoiding some inflammatory foods such as peanuts, which are especially bad for the joints.

2015 Until this point I was doing very well, albeit with ups and downs, using the strategies I had learnt over the years.

2018-19 I started having problems with my neck. I went to see a physio again who recommeded a few exercises. You must know me and exrcises by now... I followed the guidance of a health professional and can confirm it works! It took about 8 months for the pains to clear completely. A few more exercises to add to my daily routine. Nowadays I am a great believer in exercises.

2020 I have had a reasonably good start this year. I am still using all the knowledge and strategies accumulated over the years, which is the subject of this book. In November I shall turn 75, and will have completed 52 years living with chronic back pain. I would also like to remind you that in 1961 the two consultants who examined me warned me to look after myself and that I might end up in a wheelchair but advised me not to loose hope and with advances in medicine there may be help in the future. Their vision proved correct and I had a fusion operation in 1989. I intend to keep applying the PMA (Positive Mental Attititude) strategy in life come what may.

I would like to end by saying that this has not been an easy journey, in fact at times it was very hard. I have had many limitations such as not being able to do any sports, not being able to go for long walks, not being able to do many other physical activities like DIY, and so on. But by accepting my limitations and not overdoing it, I am able to live a reasonably normal life. There have been many positives along this long journey too. Not many people who know me, realise the struggles I experience, because my two battles; the physical battle and the mental battle; are invisible. Only a very few people close to me are aware that doctors predicted in 1961 that I might end up in a wheelchair.

Rounding things up, there have been many positives along this journey, many decisions, strategies, and actions taken to get me to where I am.

My Daily Action Plan

1.- Exercise – 45 minutes before I get up in the morning
2.- Medication
3.- Positive Mental Attitude- three things to eliminate from my mind: worry, hate and fear. I need to replace them with: joy, love and feeling safe. There are other negative feelings to avoid, such as frustration, anger, and so on. Worry creates anxiety which can lead to depression; hatred creates bitterness and resentment leading to feeling unloved, and fear creates a negative attitude which can lead to isolation and loneliness.
4.- Pace myself, resting when necessary.

5.- Good General Health:
  - Healthy eating
  - Socialise – interact with people, family and friends.
  - Keep active – physically as well as mentally
  - Keep a healthy weight (I ask my doctor)
  - Drink plenty of pure water.

6.- Heel Insole Cushions – I can't walk without them.

7.- Posture – bear in mind the Alexander Technique. Good posture is essential.

8.- Relaxation – or prayer and meditation

9.- Activate endorphins – either by doing: exercises, having a hot shower, with music, having a good laugh or making love.

10.- Use the Cold and Heat Treatment – as and when I need it.

11.- Use any of the distraction techniques- as and when I need to.

I hope you can get something positive and useful out of all these ideas, strategies and general knowledge. I really hope something will suit you with your specific condition. Whatever you decide to do, always consult your doctor or other trusted health professional. What worked for me might not work for you, but there are so many ideas and strategies here to safely try, with no danger of having set backs, side effects or injuries, you just have to be sensible. Thank you for reading this book. Best wishes.

APPENDICES

Appendix 1

Stretching Exercises

Flexibility or stretching exercises can be very beneficial. A few minutes each day will help you to improve the range of movement in your joints, help to decrease the risk of injury during exercise, and reduce stress. Stretching and breathing exercises help to improve your mood and lower your stress level.

Do the following exercises standing straight, ideally as soon as you get out of bed every morning. Perseverance is essential.

- Full body roll – Stand tall and extend your arms upwards towards the ceiling; then relax your arms by bringing them down, bend the upper body forward slightly and let your arms hang down and relax. Bend down as far as you can, keeping your knees bent to protect your back. Hold this position, continuing to breath for 5 to 10 seconds, then slowly roll back up and relax. Repeat this 3 times, after a few weeks you can slowly increase the number of repeats to 5, then later 10.
- Crescent moon stretches – stand tall and extend your arms up as before, then gently curve the body sideways into the shape of a

crescent moon very gently to the left and then to the right. Start by doing this 3 times. As with the above exercise after a few weeks you can increase the repeats.

- Neck and shoulders stretches – In an upright seated or preferably standing position, gently tilt the chin towards your chest then hold this position for 10 seconds, you should feel a gentle release in the back of the neck, then gently bring your chin up again. Repeat this 3 times; later increase it as above.

  The second exercise: sitting or standing up straight, maintaining your shoulders and neck straight gently move your head forward keeping your shoulders still, hold for 3 seconds, then return to the starting position, repeat 3 times. Next, push your head back with your chin down and hold for 2 seconds before returning to the starting position, and relax. Increase as above.

A third gentle exercise: move or roll your head very slowly sideways first to your left and hold for 3 seconds, return to the starting position, then roll right in a similar fashion and hold for 3 seconds, returning to the normal position. Again 3 times and increase as above. Do these neck exercises very gently, taking care not to over do it.

- Chest open and stretch – In a standing position, clasp your hands together behind your back . Feel the front of your chest open and then stretch. Hold for 5 to 10 seconds, then relax. Repeat this 5 times. Increase as above.

The following exercises can be done lying on the bed:

- Lift and stretch your arms as if trying to touch the ceiling, stretch out your fingers, hold for 5 seconds; then bring arms down to the start position, and relax. Repeat this 3 times, a couple of weeks later increase to 5, later to 10.

* Extend your legs focussing on your feet, keeping your feet at 90 degrees, relax your feet for a minute. Extend and stretch one leg away from you, hold it for 3 seconds, then bring it back to the starting position, and relax. Then do the same with the other leg. Repeat 3 times. Now a similar exercise, but this time relax your feet for a minute, then move only your toes backwards and forwards, for 3 seconds, bring them back to the starting position, and relax. Repeat 3 times. Next bring your toes towards you, hold for 3 seconds, and return to the starting position, and relax. Repeat 3 times.

***

Appendix 2

Arthritis – How to keep your joints healthy

1. Keep moving your joints – Many people with joint pain or arthritis believe/think that by being physically active or doing exercise their pain will increase or cause more damage. In fact, movement/exercise eases joint stiffness, reduces pain, strengthens the muscles surrounding the joints and helps maintain a healthy weight.

2. Maintain your ideal weight – carrying excess body weight adds stress to our joints. Check with your GP or other Health Professional what your ideal weight is.
3. Low impact exercises – According to the arthritis Foundation, low-impact exercises are very beneficial to joints, for instance, swimming, social sports such as walking, cycling, golf, bowls and so on.
4. Strengthening your muscles around joints – The muscles that support our joints work in combination with tendons and ligaments therefore must be kept as strong as possible.

Personal experience – This is exactly what I did when I had arthritic pains in nearly all my joints. I asked my GP to refer me to a physio, learnt all the exercises for my joints, and did them diligently every day and persevered, as mentioned above.

Be careful and disciplined, pacing your workouts and not overdoing it.

5. An anti-inflammatory diet may be beneficial – According to the Arthritis Foundation incorporating more foods from the Mediterranean diet may help to control inflammation – foods that are rich in anti-oxidants and phytochemicals.

   Foods recommended are: fruits, especially berries; any raw or cooked vegetables; beans and legumes; whole and cracked grains; healthy fats such as nuts, avocado and virgin olive oil; whole soy foods like tofu; fish and sea food: spices, herbs and herbal teas; red wine and dark chocolate (in moderation).

Foods to avoid are: frozen or packaged ready-meals; packaged snack foods; desserts, baked goods, ice cream; fatty foods, fried foods; soda or soft drinks; foods made with white flour or sugar. Margarine and foods made with omega-6 oils; red meat and dairy products must only be enjoyed in moderation.

***

Appendix 3

Breathing exercises – Step by step technique for use at home

1. Find a warm quiet place. Lie on a rug or sit comfortably in a well supported chair. Reduce outside noises if possible.
2. Wear loose clothing and remove glasses and shoes. Lie on your back with your head supported (6-7 cms off the floor ie. a couple of books), and your arms and legs straight and slightly apart.
3. Breathe in and out deeply for 3 breaths and imagine you are loosening the tension. Then breathe normally.
4. Close your eyes and keep focussed. You are going to work on each major muscle group starting from your feet. As you tighten and relax, learn to recognise the difference between tension and relaxation. Hold each contraction for 3 seconds breathing in, return to the starting position breathing out, and relax. Reapeat 3 times with a short break in between each time.
5. Now draw your feet towards your body maintaining straight legs, hold the contraction (tension) for 3 seconds breathing in, return to the starting position breathing out, and relax. With this release

you will feel the reduction in tension. Repeat this 3 times with a short break.

6. Point your toes as much as you can away from your body, breathing in and feel the tension in your calf muscles; hold for 3 seconds, return to the starting position, and relax. Repeat this 3 times.
7. Relaxing your thigh muscles. Lie on your back on a comfortable surface (ie a foam mat or bed) have your head up about 6-7 cms (ie books or pillow/cushion). Bring your knees up towards you keeping your feet flat on the mat.

   <u>This is the most recommended position for resting your back.</u> Now you are ready to exercise your thigh muscles. Hold your left leg with both hands just below your knee, bring the knee towards your left shoulder trying to touch it and breathing in; hold for 3 seconds and relax breathing out. Repeat with your right leg.

   Repeat 3 times. Feel the tension when you bring your knee towards the shoulder and feel the reduction of tension when you go back to the resting position.

8. Tense your buttocks by squeezing them hard together; hold for 5 seconds; and relax.

   Repeat this 3 times.

9. Tense your abdomen muscles by bringing your stomach inwards for 3 seconds and relax. Now tense your abdomen muscles again but this time push outwards, hold for 3 seconds, and relax.

10. At this point, a few deep breaths will help. Breathe in slowly, then slowly release your breath while focusing on all the parts of your body you have been working out, and make sure your body feels steady, warm and relaxed.
11. Now concentrate on your back. Lying down with your arms next to your body arch your spine towards your stomach, breathing in pushing with your legs and your arms, away from the flat mat. Hold for 3 seconds and relax.

    Warning – Avoid this exercise if you have any back problems.

12. In a standing position, move your shoulders backwards to expand your chest, breathing in, hold for 3 seconds, and relax.
13. Lying down and your arms at your side, work your hands and lower arms by making tight fists; hold for 3 seconds, and relax. As you clench your fists for the second time, raise your arms slightly keeping your elbows straight and feel the tension in your forearms, hold for 3 seconds, and relax.
14. Still lying down, work your upper arms by bringing your hands across your body close to your chest, hold for 3 seconds, and relax by bringing your arms back down next to your body, and with the palms of your hands facing upwards.
15. Next clench your jaw by clamping your teeth together; hold for 3 seconds and let go, so your mouth is slightly open.
16. To work your facial muscles press your lips together; hold and relax. Push your tongue hard to the roof of your mouth; hold for 3 seconds, then let it drop to the floor of your mouth.

17. Finally relax your forehead and scalp. Frown hard and pull your forehead down; hold for 3 seconds and let go so that your face feels loose.

***

Appendix 4

Listening Exercise

1. Sit in an upright comfortable chair with your back well supported.
2. Now notice all the sounds that you can hear, loud sound, sounds far away. Just hear them, don't even try to name them.
3. Notice fainter sounds, and sounds which are nearer. Just listen, become aware ot them.
4. Can you hear the sound of your own heartbeat? It may be faint, but that's your own rhythm of life.
5. And the sound of silence in your state of meditation or prayer; the silence within yourself...
6. Just listen for a few minutes. Once you get the hang of it, you will find it very relaxing.

***

Appendix 5

Imagination Exercise

Withdraw in your imagination to some place in which you have experienced happiness in the past.

Once you have chosen this place take some time recapturing every detail. Use each of your imaginative senses for this:

* see the objects in the place, their colours, their shape...
* hear every sound, both loud and quiet...
* touch, taste and smell if that is possible... until the place becomes as fully present to you as possible.

– What are you doing?
– What are you feeling?
– What are you thinking?

After being in this place for 5 minutes, come back to the present situation.

– What are you feeling now?
– Stay with this for 2 or 3 minutes.

Return again to the imagined place?

– And what do you feel now?

Return again to the present situation. Move between the two.

– Notice your feelings

Try to recapture something of that experience and bring it into the present.

***

Appendix 6

Top 5 Essential Oils especially for Arthritis

1. Ginger - Is an amazing healing agent – contains chemicals with analgesic and anti-inflammatory effects on the body.
2. Turmeric – Contains curcumin known as a great anti-inflammatory. A good easy to prepare suggestion is 'turmeric tea'.

   Ingredients:
   1 cup of coconut milk / 1 cup of water / 1 tablespoon of ghee / 1 tablespoon of honey / 1 teaspoon of turmeric (powder or grated root).

   Preparation:
   1. Pour coconut milk and water into the saucepan – warm for 2 minutes.
   2. Add in butter, honey and turmeric powder – warm for a further 2 minutes.
   3. Stir and pour into a cup.

3. Frankincense – Reduces inflammation on pain-related conditions that affect the muscles, joints and tendons.

4. Myrrh oil – Has anti-inflammatory properties, often used in tandem with frankincense to treat arthritis. A study published in SCIENTIFIC REPORTS shows that frankincense and myrrh combined are highly effective in the treatment of inflammatory diseases.

5. Orange – Orange oil has been researched and a 2009 study published in the European Journal of Medical Research reported that * *orange oil was the most highly effective of those studied, which in turn makes it a great essential oil for arthritis treatment.*

Best supplement sources

- Marine or fish oils
- Blackcurrent seed oil
- Flaxseed (linseed) oil
- Evening primrose oil
- Borage starflower oil

Best food sources

- Oily fish (tuna, mackerel, herring)
- Dark green leafy vegetables
- Sunflower and sesame seeds
- Pumpkin seeds, oats, wheat and rice
- Peas, lentils and beans.

***

Appendix 7

The Various Benefits of Drinking Pure Water

1. Increases brain power and provides energy - Your brain is made of 73% water. Drinking plenty of water will help you think, focus concentrate and stay alert. Your energy level will improve as well. According to research, "Being dehydrated by just 2% impairs performance in tasks that require attention and immediate memory skills". Dehydration can affect your mood, and reduce cognitive and motor skills. It raises pain sensitivity, and can affect your memory.
2. Promotes healthy weight management and weight loss – Water aids in the removal of fat by-products and helps you feel full. It can also improve your metabolism.
3. Flush out toxins – Water helps your body flush out waste through sweat and urination. This also prevents kidney stones and protects you from urinary tract infections.
4. Improves your complexion – About 60 to 65 % of your body weight comes from water, according to Iowa State University. Although the percentage of water in the human body varies by age and gender. The average adult male will have 60% of water; the average adult female will have 55%; children will have 65% and infants 75%. So dehydration will harm your skin. Dehydration can make your skin go dry, tight and flaky. Drinking plenty of water helps to moisturise your skin, will keep it soft and removes wrinkles.
5. Boosts your immune system – Drinking plenty of water helps you have a healthy immune system.

6. Prevents headaches – One of the most common symptoms of dehydration is headaches. And water helps to relieve, even prevent, headaches often caused by dehydration.
7. Prevents cramps and sprains – It is well established that dehydration leads to cramping. Water acts as a natural lubricant for your muscles and joints, and as a result you will be more flexible.
8. Helps regulate your body-temperature – It replenishes your body cooling system – sweat. Your body needs enough water to properly regulate body-temperature through perspiration.
9. Prevents backaches – The bones of your vertebrae are supported by discs; and the central nucleous of each disc is made of water. A lack of water can compromise these discs leading to back pain.
10. Lemon water – If you add lemon to water it is even better. Lemons are a great source of vitamin C, which is known to boost the immune system, prevent disease, fight the common cold and protect cells.
11. Improves the health of your heart – Research has shown a link between coronary heart disease and water consumption. Water maintains the proper viscosity of blood and plasma.

This is also my experience. When I went to see my cardiologist (I have been suffering from angina and atrial fibrilation/arrhythmia for quite some time) in Januay 2018, he asked me how much water I was drinking and I admitted that I was not drinking much at all (only in the summer or when it is very hot). He told me I should drink a lot more water . I greatly increased my water intake and the result after a few months was amazing. I felt so much better.

What is the Function of Water in the Body?

Water serves multiple purposes:

- It is the primary building block of cells.
- It acts as an insulator, regulating internal body temperatures, plus the body uses perspiration and respiration to regulate temperature.
- Water is needed to metabolise proteins and carbohydrates used as food. It is the primary component of saliva used to digest carbohydrates and aid to swallowing food.

- Water insulates the brain, spinal cord, organs and fetus. It acts as a shock absorber.
- Water is used to flush waste and toxins from the body via urine.
- Water is the principal solvent in the body. It dissolves minerals, soluble vitamins and certain nutrients.
- Water carries oxygen and nutrients to all cells, which results in properly functioning systems.

***

Appendix 8

Avoiding Inflammatory Foods

Consumption of inflammatory foods makes arthritis and chronic back pain worse. These are some of the worst foods you should be aware of:

- Salty foods – The recommended daily limit is 1500 miligrams, yet most people eat more than double at an average of 3400mg. a day.

When your kidneys can't eliminate salt fast enough, it accumulates in your bloodstream. Since salt holds water, blood vessels swell with the extra blood volume. As blood vessels expand, they may place pressure on your joints tissue and cause pain.

- Sugar – In 2015 the World Health Organisation (WHO), called on countries around the world to "reduce their daily intake of free sugars to less than 10% of their total energy intake for adults and children. The problem is that sugar is hidden in many foods and fizzy drinks. The average 12-ounce can of soda contains around 8 ounces of sugar. So it only takes 4 x 12-ounce cans to equal ¼ pound of sugar. Always check the labels.
- Alternatives to sugar – Alternative to sugar (artificial sweeteners) can cause inflammation reaction in those who are sensitive to it, and should also be avoided.
- Alcohol – Alcohol contains high amounts of sugar and it is also a diuretic. It blocks the release of anti-diuretic hormones (ADH), which the kidneys need to reabsorb water for proper function.
- Refined grains – Processed grains, like white flour and corn (found in crackers, pastries and other snack foods) have a higher glycemic index than unprocessed grains and can cause inflammation.
- Grain-Fed Beef – Conventional beef comes from cows fed from the same grains and are likely to cause inflammation. It is high in Omega-6 fatty acids, which can trigger inflammation. A healthier balance of Omega-3 fatty acids is found in grass-fed beef, as well as grass-fed chickens (and eggs).

Food Best Choices

- Fruits - red, blue and purple berries, grapes, pomegranates, plums, cherries, oranges, peaches, nectarines, apples and pears, papaya, apricots and persimmons.
- Vegetables – all are good, especially dark leafy greens, broccoli, cabbage, Brussel sprouts, cauliflower, carrots, onions, garlic, peas, pumpkins, avocados, and sweet potatoes.
- Beans and legumes – Anasazi, adzuki, black beans, chick peas, black-eyed beans, peas and lentils.
- Pasta- Go for quality over quantity – organic pasta, rice noodles, bean thread noodles, wholewheat and buckwheat noodles, as well as spinach pasta.
- Whole and cracked grains – sorghum, millet, brown and wild rice, quinoa and couscous.
- Healthy fats in nuts and seeds – All nuts and seeds are very similar in terms of nutrient content: They are high in mono-unsaturated and poly-unsaturated fats; low in saturated fats; free of dietary cholesterol; high in dietary fibre; and rich in vitamin E, B6, niacin and folate (containing lots of minerals such as magnesium, zinc, calcium, selenium, phosphorous and potassium). These are: walnuts, Brazil nuts, almonds, hazelnuts, pecans and others; also flaxseeds, hemp seeds, chia seeds. Also mono-unsaturated fats are found in avocados, olives and extra virgin olive oil.

  Warning: Do not give nuts to children under the age of 5, as they may choke on them. In regard to allergies, nuts can trigger life-threatening reactions in people with a nut allergy.`

- Fish and sea-food – They are packed with anti-inflammatory Omega-3 fats: salmon, herring, sardines, mackerel and black cod.
- Selenium-rich foods – Selenium is a powerful anti-oxidant mineral (anti-oxidants protect the cells from damage). It plays a key role in the metabolism (turning food into energy). Benefits: it may help reduce the risk of cetain cancers; it may protect you against heart disease; it can help prevent mental decline (ie. Alzehimer's disease); it can help with proper functioning of your thyroid gland; it can boost your immune system; and it may reduce asthma symptoms.
- Good sources on selenium include: Brazil nuts, fish (especially tuna and shellfish), ham, enriched foods (pastas, whole wheat breads, whole wheat cereals), lean pork, lean beef, turkey, lean chicken breast, cottage cheese, eggs, sunflower seeds, baked beans, mushrooms, oatmeal (whole oats) spinach, milk, yogurt, lentils, cashew nuts, bananas, whole grains (whole wheat flour, bulgur or cracked wheat, whole cornmeal, brown rice), whole oats (whole grain oat grouts, steel cut oats and thick oats), whole wheat (cereals, breads, pastas, crackers, muffins and cakes).
- Spices – turmeric, ginger, garlic, basil, cinnamon, rosemary and thyme.

***

Appendix 9

Foods to Avoid with Arthritis, Joint and Back Pain

If you suffer from arthitis or any other condition with pain to your joints or the spine these are the inflammatory foods you need to avoid:

- Fried and processed foods – Studies show that decreasing the amount of fried and processed foods eaten can reduce inflammation and help restore the body's natural defences.
- Sugars and refined carbs – cut down (or stop) eating sweets, processed foods, white flour baked goods and fizzy drinks.
- Dairy products – may contribute to arthritis pain due to the type of protein they contain. Try getting your protein from vegetables like spinach, nuts, tofu, beans, lentils and quinoa.
- Alcohol and tobacco – they both can lead to various health problems, some may affect your joints. If you smoke, you are at risk of developing rheumatoid arthritis.
- Corn oil – many baked goods and snacks contain corn or other oils high in Omega-6 fatty acids, which may trigger inflammation. According to the Mayo Clinic (USA), some studies have found that fish oil, which contain Omega-3, may help with joint pain relief.
- Salt and preservatives – many foods contain excessive salt and other preservatives to promote longer shelf-life. Too much salt may result in inflammation to your joints and spine. Less salt may help.

Read on to see alternatives to salt.

- Cinnamon – sprinkle some on top of your oatmeal instead of brown sugar.
- Turmeric – sprinkle some on eggs and chicken.
- Oregano – have it with sauces, proteins and grains.
- Black pepper and cayenne – have it with soups, grilled veggies or meats.
- Kelp granules – are sea vegetables and an excellent salt alternative; it can be added to grains and soups.
- Citrus fruits – these are a very good salt alternatives, plus a great source of vitamin C. Squeeze a lemon, orange or grapefruit over salads, seafood and marinades.
- Sunflower seeds – they can be sprinkled on just about any meal...
- Vinegar – add it to sauces, marinades, dressings and salads. Try different types of flavoured vinegars
- Red wine – add to sauces or gravy; or as a marinade for meats and veggies. You can also add to soups, pasta sauces, stews and even salads (instead of vinegar).
- Spices in general – be adventurous and try more spices as alternatives to salt. We have mentioned a few, and here you have more: mint, rosemary, nutmeg, basil, chives , coriander, cumin, ginger, parsley, paprika, and thyme.

***

Appendix 10

The Pituitary Gland

The pituitary gland is a small pea-sized gland that plays a major role in regulating vital body functions and general well-being. It is referred to as the body's 'master gland' because it controls the activity of most other hormone-secreting glands. It is a bony hollow in the base of the skull, underneath the brain and behind the bridge of the nose.

It secretes a variety of hormones into the bloodstream which acts as messengers to transmit information from the pituitry gland to distant cells, regulating their activity.

The pituitary gland produces *prolactin,* which acts on the breast to induce milk production during lactation. It also secretes hormones that act on the adrenal glands, thyrod glands, ovaries and testes, which in turn produce other hormones.

Through secretion of hormones, the pituitary gland controls your *metabolism:* growth, sexual maturation, reproduction, blood pressure, and many other vital physical functions and processes.

***

Appendix 11

The Benefits of Making Love

There are many emotional and psychological benefits from making love which are strongly linked to overall quality of life. Some of these include the following benefits:

- Happiness – According to a 2015 study carried out in Asia, more sex and higher quality intercourse increases pleasure/happiness (although unwanted sex lowers it).
- Stress Relief – Our bodies secrete CORTISOL and ADRENALINE (epinephrine) within the anxiety response. These are hormones that work as key players in the body's stress response. These hormones can lead to fatigue, hypertension, high blood pressure and more.
- Improves Mood – There are a number of chemicals our bodies release during love making that can affect how we feel. During sex our brains release endorphins (see above page 107), a 'feel good' chemical that can reduce stress and feelings of depression. Orgasm leads to the release of yet another hormone, PROLACTIN that can help with a better sleep. Love making can boost self-esteem and lower feelings of insecurity, leading to a more positive attitude.
- Better Immune Function - Being more sexually active also has positive effects on immune function and make it less likely to get a cold or flu.
- Cardiac Effects – Sexual activity has been linked with lower systolic blood pressure; it is thought that sexual acitivity helps dilate blood vessels, increasing the delivery of oxigen and nutrients to the cells of the body while reducing blood pressure.

- Brain Effects – A 2018 study looking at over 6,000 adults found that making love more often was associated with better memory performance in adults ages 50 and older.
- Relationship Benefits – Making love often can benefit you and your parrtner individually, but it can also help you both in other ways. Making love in a monogamous relationship can increase your level of commitment and help you connect emotionally. The release of oxytocin can contribute to bonding and greater emotional intimacy.
- Reduces Pain – The endorphins mentioned above do more than create a feeling of well-being and calm, it can also reduce pain.

***

Appendix 12

Certain Foods that Help to Release Endorphins

You probably know that when eating certain foods there is the tendency to make you feel better. These are foods that contain certain nutrients that encourage the release of endorphins.

– Dark chocolate - Research shows that dark chocolate has lots of health benefits, and can heighten sensitivity and even produce euphoric effects through the release of endorphins. It is known to reduce the stress hormone cortisol. It has high quantities of phenols, which are anti-oxidants that can boost people's mood.
– Strawberries – Are a super-food: 1. They are a rich source of anti-oxidants (vitamin C). 2. they support the immune sysytem. 3.

Strawberries may help with blood sugar regulation. 4. They may have antimicrobial effects. 5. They may improve heart health. Numerous studies have found that their high content of berry anthocyanins may play a role in reducing inflammation and oxidative stress, blood pressure and even improving our cholesterol profile. Strawberries are a smart fruit choice for diabetics as they have a lower glycemic index (40) than many other fruits.

- Nuts and seeds - They not only contain healthy fats, but they are also rich in vitamin B, protein and selenium. Brazil nuts and sunflower seeds are known as the richest source of selenium, known to have positive mood-influencing properties.
- Grapes - Are high in endorphin-producing vitamin C and also a good source of potassium. They are a good source of antioxidants that can help support health.
- Apples – Produce a calming effect and give us energy.
- Asparagus – Contain high levels of tryptophan, a key ingredient in making serotonin that promotes calming and relaxation. Serotonin in the brain helps prevent depression and anxiety.
- Bananas – Are full of potassium and tryptophan, a brain chemical that regulates your mood. They are also a good source of B vitamin folate. A banana a day provides enough vitamin B6, which helps regulate mood and keep people feeling calm and relaxed.
- Beans – Are good for the heart and the mind. The selenium in them gives you more energy. Beans can boost the mood and keep you happier.
- Brown rice – Can naturally boost serotonin levels that provide stress relief.
- Coffee – A mood enhancer which can lower depression.
- Eggs – According to the American Journal of Clinical Nutrition,

eggs are high in choline that helps boost memory. They are also a good source of vitamin D which helps fight depression. According to the NHS (UK), eating one egg a day may lower the risk of stroke, but not the risk of heart disease. This issue has been debated for years: Eggs, which contain cholesterol, were thought to increase risk of heart disease by raising cholesterol levels, though recent studies show that cholesterol in food has little impact on the level of cholesterol in your blood (most of the blood is made by the liver).

- Ginseng – Helps combat fatigue and stress as it balances the release of stress hormones. It may also help release endorphins.
- Greek yogurt – The calcium in Greek yogurt alerts the brain to release feel good chemicals. Insufficient calcium can contribute to irritability, anxiety and depression.
- Mushrooms – Are very high in vitamin D which helps reduce irritability, anxiety and depression.
- Oranges – Are a great source of vitamin C which also helps to reduce irritability, anxiety and depression.
- Sea food – Omega-3 fatty acids in fish increases serotonin and dopamine levels which produce hormones that make you feel good. For instance salmon is full of Omega-3 fatty acids.
- Spinach – Alliviates depression and reduces fatigue due to its folic acid content.
- Tomatoes – Lycopene in tomatoes is an extremely potent antioxidant that helps keep at bay inflammation which causes depression, and it reduces stress.
- Turmeric – The curcumin in turmeric helps fight depression by increasing serotonin and dopamine levels.
- Quinoa – A carbohydrate that can help prevent depression and anxiety by increasing levels of serotonin in the brain. It also contains

a flavonoid, quercetin, that helps eliminate anxiety and depression.

- Walnuts – Their high content of antioxidants, vitamins and minerals, help improve the mood. They also contain a large amount of Omega-3 that gives the brain the amount of endorphins that keep people in a good mood.
- Water – We have referred to water in Appendix 7, but in this section we need to mention it once again because there is a link between water and stress reduction. Every organism in our body including the brain needs water to function properly. Being dehydrated can lead to stress. Hydration can calm and boost your mood as well.
- Wine - Drinking wine in moderation, especially red wine, has been found to improve emotional well-being as it reduces stress and anxiety, and helps you to relax. Excess intake of alcoholic drinks, including wine, can lead to other health problems.

What are antioxidants? - They are compounds produced in the body and also found in foods. They help defend cells from damage caused by potentially harmful molecules known as 'free radicals'. Selenium works alongside antioxidants to clear your system of free radicals.

The richest source of antioxidants are (ORAC value for antioxidants):

- Black raspberries – 19,220
- Elderberries – 14,697
- Blueberries – 9621
- Cranberries – 9090
- Black currants – 7957
- Black diamond plums – 7581
- Blackberries – 5905
- Pomegranates – 4479

- Strawberries – 4302
- Red apples – 4275
- Avocado - 1992

Cacao and dark chocolate; pecan nuts; artichokes; kale; broccoli; red cabbage; beans; beetroot; spinach and many spices, such as: cinnamon, ginger, cloves, turmeric, chilli and garlic are also high in antioxidants.

***

Appendix 13

Drumming and Endorphins

The findings of a University of Oxford study show that participatory music, such as drumming, triggers the release of endorphins, increasing the pain threshold.

Several scientific studies have shown that playing drums can provide a measurable impact on stress relief, cardio health and general happiness.

In his book "The Healing Power of the Drum", psychotherapist Robert Lawrence Friedman shares an interview with Barry Quinn, a clinical psychologist specialising in neuro feedback and stress management. Quinn says "drumming can change a person's brain wave patterns by prompting the release of alpha waves, which are associated with a general feeling of wellbeing and euphoria".

Drumming has a therapeutic value, providing the emotional and physical benefits collectively known as " drummer's high", an endorphin rush that can only be stimulated by playing music rather than simply listening to it. Oxford psychologists found that the endorphin-filled drumming increases positive emotions and leads people to work together in a more cooperative fashion.

The benefits of playing drums are:

- It releases endorphins in your brain that creates happiness and euphoria and it is fun.
- Boosts your immune system - Studies show it can create illness-killing cells which can protect your body.
- Reduces stress and lowers blood pressure.
- Brings positivity by helping people express and address emotional trauma.
- Great workout – Good exercise, a physical activity which improves reflexes and stimulates the brain.
- Improves coordination as it is an instrument that requires more coordination than any other.
- Develops creative skills – You can play drums in a creative way, new rhythms, new sounds, etc.
- Sharpens concentration, especially when playing with other musicians and other instruments.
- Helps you connect with self and others – It creates a sense of working in a group and coordinating with others.

- Helps improve social skills – It help you socialise with other people and improves interpersonal skills as you get to learn with others.

***

Appendix 14

Musical Interventions in Music Therapy (MT)

For understanding the kind of musical interventions which may be used in music therapy, the following is a list provided by the Canadian Association for Music Therapy (CAMT).

- Singing – Improves articulation, rhythm, and breath control. It reduces anxiety and fear.
- Playing instruments – Improves gross and fine motor coordination. Enhances cooperation, attention, and provides leadership opportunities and other participant roles. Develops an increase in well-being and self-esteem.
- Rhythmic based activities – facilitates and improves range of motion, joint mobility, agility strength, balance, coordination, consistency and relaxation. Rhythm and beat (ie. drumming) are important in "priming the motor areas of the brain, in regulating autonomic processes such as breathing and heart rate".
- Improvising – Offers a creative, non-verbal means of expressing thoughts and feelings. It is non-judgemental, easy to approach, and requires no previous musical training.

- Composing - facilitates the sharing of feelings, ideas and experiences. Lyric discussions and song writing can help individuals deal with painful memories, trauma, abuse, and express socially unacceptable feelings and thoughts.
- Listening – Helps to develop cognitive skills such as attention and memory. In situations where cognitive perceptions are compromised, such as in early to mid stage dementia, listening can provide a sense of a familiarity and increase orientation to reality.

Music Therapy Intervention	Benefit	Pain Perceptions
Singing	Articulation, breathing	***Catharsis** (reduces anxiety) = less pain
Playing instruments	Increased well-being feeling of being a part of something/self-expession	Well-being = less pain
Rhythmic based activities	Regulate breathing and heart rate Relaxation	Relaxation = less pain
Improvising	Contact/expression Possible release of endorphins	***Catharsis** = less pain-related Endorphins = body's natural pain killers
Composing	Sharing feeling, experiences possible release of endorphins (stimulation of limbic system)	***Catharsis** = less pain-related Endorphins – body's natural pain killers
Listening	Stimulate memories, elicit emotions (stimulation of limbic system)	Override pain subjective experience = less pain-related

www.music therapy.ca

* **Catharsis =** the process of releasing, and thereby providing relief from strong or repressed emotions.

***

Appendix 15

Progressive Muscle Relaxation

Make yourself comfortable. Wearing loose clothing lie down on something firm but comfortable, such as a foam mat or mattress. Raise your head slightly using a pillow or cushion. Close your eyes.

Take a deep breath, filling your lungs and breathing all the way down to your abdomen. Hold for 3 seconds... Breath out slowly let the air out through slightly parted lips. As you breath out release as much tension as possible. Let your muscles feel heavy and then relax them, letting your body go floppy.

Concentrate on the muscles of your feet and calves. Keeping your legs straight pull your toes toward your knees, and focus on the tension... Release and relax... Now point your toes away from you and focus on the tension... Release and relax... and feel the warmth.

Feel the muscles of your thighs and buttocks totally floppy and then tighten them up. Hold and focus on the tension... Let go and relax.

Now tense the muscles in your abdomen and chest... Hold for 3 seconds... Release and relax. Take a deep breath or two, breathing all the way down to the abdomen slowly, letting it expand outwardly. As you breathe out, allow all the tension to flow out.

This time, focus on your fingers and arms. Stretch your fingers out straight, tense them and tighten your arm muscles. Hold for 3 seconds...

Relax and feel the tension flowing away.

Press your shoulder blades together, tightening the muscles in your shoulders and neck. Hold for 3 seconds... Relax... You should feel your muscles warmer amd more relaxed.

Grimace or 'pull a face' to tighten the muscles of your face and head. Focus on the tension around your eyes and in your jaw. Hold for 3 seconds... and relax.

By foccusing on your breathing during your muscle tensing and relaxing you will be feeling the difference it makes.

Now, take a deep breath, breathing in slowly all the way down to your abdomen and slowly out. You should be feeling very relaxed. Take another deep breath in the same way... and relax.

Finally, take one last breath... And RELAX. If you doze off during these exercises you're doing an excellent job!

***

Appendix 16

Centring Prayer

Most religions use some form of prayer. As mentioned above, prayer is a way of talking, listening and spending precious time with your

God. It is a time when you can express or share your feelings, wants and needs comfortably. You can pray corporately, as in a church or temple, or privately. You may want to give thanks, ask for help or forgiveness and praise your God. There are very different types of prayer but you might want to try Centring Prayer, which is similar to some types of meditation.

Choose a sacred or special word or phrase – something like Lord, Father, Mother, Abba, Omm, love, peace, shalom or something significant to you to express your intention for the centring prayer. Avoid doing this after a meal. Find a quiet and comfortable place to either lie down or sit. Relax your whole body and close your eyes. Let go of any thoughts going on in your mind (put them to one side for the duration of this process) and focus on your sacred/special word or phrase all the time. When youf finish your prayer, stay in silence with your eyes closed for at least a couple of minutes, or as long as you wish.

Just allow yourself to be aware of any sensations you may have experienced for a short time, and return to your sacred/special word.

If you are doing this for the first time, start by doing it every couple of days or even every day if you can, so you get into a routine. Later, you may want to progress to twice a day; it's a very personal choice. Setting times of the day will help create a routine. If you persevere you will experience positive results.

***

Appendix 17

Mindfulness Meditation

The main purpose of meditation is to quieten your mind. It is very useful for people with long-term conditions. It is easily achievable and can help manage pain, stress, tiredness and shortness of breath.

All you need to have is a quiet place and five minutes. You can sit on a chair with your feet flat on the ground, and place your hands on your lap. If you prefer, you could sit on the floor. The important thing is that you feel comfortable.

What is fundamental in mindfulness meditation is to concentrate on your breathing. Diaphragmatic (or belly) breathing (see below) is the best approach.

Breath in slowly, hold your breath for 3 seconds; then breath out slowly, concentrating all the time on your breathing. Some people tend to allow their minds wander and think of other things. When you realise this, refocus and concentrate on your breathing.

It is likely that you might get positive results fairly soon, but the experts say it requires practice. They advise 5 minutes a day to start with, then building up to 15, then later on to 30 minutes a day, 4 or 5 times a week.

Diaphragmatic breathing – Diaphragmatic breathing is also known as breathing control or belly breathing. It strengthens the breathing muscles; and with more efficient muscles you can put less energy into your breathing. Again it requires practice.

Remember diaphragmatic breathing wil lhelp you contol your breathing with less effort. Here are the 4 steps you need to help you learn to control your breathing:

1. Lie on your back with a pillow under your head and one under your knees (if that is comfortable for you). Put one hand on your stomach, below your breastbone, and the other hand on your upper chest. Breathe in slowly through your nose keeping your mouth closed, allowing your stomach to expand outward. As you breathe in your lungs will fill with fresh air and the hand that you have on your stomach will move upward. The hand on your chest should not move noticeably.

Now breathe out slowly through pursed lips.

2. When you feel comfortable doing this, you could place a light weight on your abdomen. This will help strengthen the muscles used to breathe in. Start with a weight of about one pound (500 grams) like a book or a bag of rice. A few weeks later you can increase the weight as your muscle strength improves.
3. You can also practice diaphragmatic breathing sitting in a chair. You need to relax your shoulders, arms, hands and chest. Put one hand on your abdomen as before and the other on your chest. Breathe in slowly through your nose as much as you can; the hand in your chest should remain still and the hand on your abdomen will move outwards. Now breathe out gently and with little effort.

4. Once you feel comfortable with this technique, you can practice it almost at any time when you are lying down, sitting or standing. This breathing technique can help strengthen and improve the coordination and efficiency of the breathing muscles, and at the same time decrease the amount of energy you use to breath.

You can also use it alongside any of the relaxation techniques mentioned in this book.

***

Appendix 18

The Origins and History of Prayer and Meditation in our World

The earliest writings to be discovered around 1500BC in India, were concerning the practice of Dhyana meditation, originating from the Vedas of Hindu traditions. The Vedas philosophy is one of the earliest known in India. The Vedas are a collection of hymns and ancient religious texts, and include liturgical material, mythological accounts, poems and prayers.

Over time meditation was developed further by the traditions of Hinduism, Jaimism and Buddhism, although the technical contexts vary in each religion.

Soon, when Buddhism was spreading through China, the writings of Vimalakirti Sutra (100BC) included meditations and enlightened wisdom practiced by the Zen (a school of Mahayana Buddhism) originated in China during the Tang dynasty. It was strongly influenced by Taoist philosophy, which included meditative practices and the idea of wisdom in silence. In the 2nd century, Dosho, a Japanese monk, travelled to China to study Buddhism. It was during this journey that Dosho learned about the process of Zen. When he returned he created a community of monks and students with the aim to teach this form of meditation in Japan.

The concept of Dhikr or Remembrance of God in Islam, is interpreted by various meditative techniques and became one of the essential elements in Sufism in the 11th and 12th centuries. In Sufism, thinking/meditating leads to knowledge and its followers practice control of breathing as well as incorporating the repetition of holy words.

Eastern Christian meditation also involves the repetition of a phrase and is traced back to the Byzantine period. Hesychasm was developed in Mount Athos, Greece and involves the repetition of Jesus prayer. This form of meditation is still being practiced today. Lectio Divina, a meditative practice developed by the Benedictine monks in the West uses different Scripture passages and is not repetitive in nature.

In Judaism the first prayer, which is recorded in the Torah and Hebrew Bible, occurred when Abraham pledged with God not to destroy the people of Sodom where his nephew Lot and other righteous people lived. King David who reigned over Israel for 40 years (1010BC – 970 BC), wrote lots of poems and prayers recorded in the Bible in the Book of Psalms. Isaac (described in the Torah as "lasuach") son of Abraham, appears in the Torah, and it is said that he was participating in some type of meditative practice. In the Book of Genesis though, Iasuach's activity is translated as meditation, yet all commentaries define his action as prayer. This is why both prayer and meditation have been considered meditative practices throughout history and still is today.

Nowadays there is a new focus on Biblical meditation, defined as "devotional practice" of pondering the words of a verse or verses of Scripture with a receptive heart. Such Biblical meditations may correspond to specific seasons such as Lent. The meditation sequence begin by a summary of the Bible reading; then suggest specific ideas for meditation and end with an appropriate prayer. The meditation could also be designed and used for specific ordinary times/moments. The Christian meditation techniques (contemplative practices) are:

- Contemplative prayer – which usually involves the silent repetition of sacred words or phrases with focus and devotion.
- Contemplative reading – or simply contemplation, which involves thinking deeply about the teachings and events in the Bible.
- Meditating with God – a silent meditation, usually preceded by contemplation or reading, in which people focus their mind, heart and soul on the presence of God.

As you can see, the origins of prayer and meditation go a long way back, and have been practiced by very old religions in our world.

General References

Books

Battison, Toni. 2005. Taking control of your pain. Age Concern Books. England.

Cole, F.; Macdonald, H; Carus, C; & Howden-Leah, H. 2005. Overcoming Chronic Pain. A self-guide using cognitive behavioural techniques. Robinson Publishers. London

Experts Patients Programme Community Interest Company (EPPCIC). 2007. Self-management of Long-term Health Conditions. Bull Publishing Company. UK.

Fordice, W.E. 1976. Behavioural Methods for Chronic Pain. Mosby Publishers. USA.

Hage, Mike. 1992. The Back Pain Book – A Self-Help Guide for Daily Relief of Neck and Low Back Pain. Peachtree Publishers. Atlanta, Georgia, USA.

Harp, David. 1992. The 3 Minute Meditator. Judy Piatkus Publishers. London

Routledge, Gavin & Hastings, Gavin. 2003. Self Help for Backs: Say Goodbye to back pain . Harper Collins Publishers. UK

Smith, Tom. 2003. Overcoming Back Pain. Sheldon Press. London.

Thomas, Richard. 1999. Alternative Answers to pain. Marshall Publishing. London.

Watson, Andrew & Drury, Nevill. 1987. Healing Music. Nature & Health Books. Australasia, co-published with Prism Press, Dorset. UK.

Weller, Stella. 2009. Back Care Basics. Octopus Publishing Group. London.

Articles

Greer, Sarah. 2008. The Effect of Music on Pain Perception.

Willet, Sarah. 2007. Runner's High. Lehigh University. Pennsylvania. USA.

Websites

www.webmd.com/guide/pain-management/types-and-classifications

www.healthline.com/health/types-of-pain

www.about.com

www.spine-health.com/.../gate-control-theory-chronic-pain

www.everydayhealth.com/pain-management/pain-treatment.aspx

www.bing.com

www.thejoint.com

www.jointpainclinic.com

www.webmd.com/arthritis/arthritis-basics

www.arthritis.org

www.nhs.uk/conditions/back-pain/causes

www.us.humankinetics.com/blogs/except/adaptive-and-maladaptive-behavior

www.healthline.com/nutrition/glucosamine#healthy-joints

www.nhs.uk/conditions/Homeopathy

www.abchomeopathy.com/herbalremedies

www.psychologytoday.com

www.en.wikipedia.org/wiki/Positive_mental_attitude

www.sanitas.com/.../breathing-exercise-for-relaxation.html

www.project-meditation.org

www.princessinthetower.org/pain-management/pacing-for-pain-management

www.alexander.ie/improveposture.html

www.en.wikipedia.org/wiki/Alexander_technique

www.nhs.uk/conditions/stress-anxiety-depression/reduce-stress

www.spine-health.com/conditions/chronic-pain/chronic-pain

www.www.spine-health.com

www.spine-health.com/blogg/14-natural-pain-relievers

www.verywellhealth.com/back-and-neck-pain-4014758

www.webmd.com/balance/stress-management

www.nhsinform.scot/healthy-living

www.webmd.com/living-healthy

www.healthline.com/health/food-nutrition

www.draxe.com/essential-oils/essential-oils-for-arthritis

www.elementalbottles.com

www.healthyandnaturalworld.com/inflammatory-foods

www.healthline.com/nutrition/selenium-benefits

www.healthline.com/health/foods-to-avoid-with-arthritis

www.draxe.com/health/what-are-endorphins

www.yourhormones.info

www.wealthline.com/health/endorphins

www.Wikipedia.com/release-endorphins

www.psychcentral.com/lib/about-oxytocin

www.cosmopolitan.com/a30333/ways-to-boost-your-endorphins

www.sciencedirect.com/topics/neuroscience/endorphins

www.rd.com/health/wellness/natural-endorphins-boosters

www.Caloriebee.com/diets/25-Endorphin-Releasing-Foods-and...

www.webmd.com/balance/guide/massage-therapy-styles-and-health...

www.medicinenet.com

www.therapy-directory.org.uk/articles/massagetherapy.htm

www.musictherapy.ca

www.musictherapy.com

www.en.wikipedia.org/wiki/Music_therapy

www.musictherapy.org/about/musictherapy

www.digitaltrends.com/music/music-drugs-brain

www.openculture.com/2015/08/the-neuroscience-of-drumming

www.healthguide.org/.../laughter-is-the-best-medicine.htm

www.topmattress.co.uk/mattress/back_pain

www.kristinemcgee.com/improve-your-wellbeing-with-a-good-mattress

www.webmd.com/sleep-disorders

www.medical-dictionary.freedictionary.com/chiropractic

www.nhs.uk/conditions/Osteopathy

www.nhs.uk/conditions/Acupuncture

www.carm.org/what-prayer

www.liveanddare.com/contemplative-prayer-and-christian-meditation

www.psychologytoday.com/us/basics/meditation

www.positivepsychology.com/history-of-meditation

www.meditationforhealthyliving.com

www.slife.org/history-of-christian-meditation

Useful Organisations

Action on Pain – Over the last 20 plus years AOP has grown to a national organisation developing a good reputation for the quality of the support and advice that it provides. There are some interesting facts: since 1998 AOP has given over 1 million booklets; answered or made over 140,000 calls on Pain Line; received and answered over 17,000 emails; covered over 24,000 miles with the mobile Information Unit; and spoken or exhibited at 159 conferences and similar events. AOP is involved in a number of projects which have the potential to help people affected by chronic pain wherever they live.

Address: Blackthorn Drive, Scarning, Norfolk NR19 2UJ.
E-mail: painline@action-on-pain.co.uk
Painline: 0345 603 1593.
www.action-on-pain.co.uk

Anxiety UK – It is a national registered charity. It is a user-led organisation run by sufferers and ex-sufferers of anxiety disorders. We provide support to people who have been diagnosed with an anxiety condition. We give confidential advice and support to anybody suffering from anxiety or stress.

Address: Nunes House, 447 Chester Road, Manchester, M16 9HA
e-mail: support@anxietyuk.org.uk
Text support service: 07537 416 905
Helpline: 03444 775 774
www.anxietyuk.org.uk

Arthritis Action – Founded in 1942, Arthritis Action is the only UK charity giving hands-on practical help to combat the pain of arthritis through self-management and lifestyle advice. We offer people with arthritis a holistic self-management approach, looking at both the physical and mental aspects of arthritis.

Address: 56 Buckingham Gate, Westminster. London SW1E 6AE
Phone: 020 3781 7120
www.arthritisaction.org.uk

Association of Reflexologists – It is a non-profit association which has been delivering excellence in reflexology for highly qualified reflexologists, healthcare providers and members of the public since 1984. If you are looking to find a reflexologist you can trust near you, we have a search facility and then contact any of our highly trained reflexologists who are insured and committed to our Code of Practice.

Address: Victoria House, Victoria Street, Taunton, Somerset TA1 3FA
e-mail: info@aor.org.uk
Tel.: 01823 321 010
www.aor.org.uk

Back Care (Registered name: The National Back Pain Association) – It was originally set up in 1968. The charity aims to significantly reduce the burden of back and neck pain, by providing information, guidance and advice to all people and organisations and those affected by such pain.

Address: Monkey Puzzle House, 69-71 Windmill Road, Sunbury-on-Thames, TW16 7DT
e-mail: info@backcare.org.uk
Tel.: 0208 977 5474
www.backcare.org.uk

Beat – Beat is the UK's leading charity supporting those affected by eating disorders and campaigning on their behalf. Founded in 1989 as the Eating Disorders Association. People with eating disorders use disorderd eating behaviour as a way to cope with difficult situations or feelings.

Address: Neat, Unit 1 Chalk Hill House, 19 Rosary Road, Norwich, Norfolk, NR1 1SZ
e-mail: media@beateatingdisorders.org.uk
Tel.: 0300 123 3355
www.beateatingdisorders.org.uk

Brain and Spine Foundation – The Brain & Spine Foundation is the only UK-wide charity providing information for everyone of the over 470 neurological disorders which affect 1 in 6 people in the UK. Our expert services are there for people at every stage, from the first symptoms, diagnosis, treatments and in the long-term.

Address: 4th Floor, CAM Mezzanine, 7-14 Great Dover Street, London, SE1 4YR
E-mail: helpline@brainandspine.org.uk
Tel.: 0808 808 1000
www.brainandspine.org.uk

British Acupuncture Association – The BAA is one of the key organisations under the unbrella of the British Acupuncture Federation (BAF). We support public choice and the ability to access the use of acupuncture by highly trained practitioners working in both the public and the independent sectors.

Address: Suite 197, 60 Water Lane, Wilmslow Cheshire, SK9 5AJ
e-mail: enquiries@britishacupunctureassociation.co.uk
Tel.: 0843 507 0123 (for the British Acupuncture Federation too)
www.britishacupunctureassociation.co.uk

British Acupuncture Council – It is the largest professional regulatory body for the practice of acupuncture. If interested to know of a registered acupuncturist contact us.

Address: 62 Jeddo Road, Acton, London, W12 9HQ
Tel.: 020 8735 0400
www.acupuncture.org.uk

British Association for Counselling and Psychotherapy – We promote the role and relevance of the counselling professionals in improving psychological well-being and mental health. We also promote and develop safe, ethical and competent practice in counselling and psychotherapy, by raising professional standards, supporting clients and dealing with complaints about poor and unethical practice. They provide a search to help you find a local counsellor or therapist.

Address: BACP, 15 St. John's Business Park, Lutterworth, Leicestershire, LE17 4HB
Tel.: 01455 883 300
www.bacp.co.uk

British Association for Music Therapy - The BAMT is the professional body for Music Therapy in the UK, providing both practitioners and non-practitioners with information, professional support and training opportunities. It is also a charity committed to promoting and raising awareness of Music Therapy and providing information to the general public.

Address: 2nd Floor, Claremont Building, 24 – 27 White Lion Street, London, N1 9PD
e-mail: info@bamt.org
Tel.: 020 7837 6100
www.bamt.org

British Chiropractic Association – Chiropractic is a regulated primary healthcare profession. The statutory regulator is the General Chiropractic Council (GCC). Straighten Up UK is an exciting programme from the BCA, designed to improve posture and help prevent back pain by promoting balance, strength and flexibility in the spine. Chiropractors are trained to diagnose, treat, manage and prevent disorders of the musculoskeletal system (bones, joints and muscles) as well as the effects these disorders can have on the nervous system and general health. If you would like to find a local chiropractor, please contact us.

Address: 59 Castle Street, Reading, RG1 7SN
e-mail: enquiries@chiropractic-uk.co.uk
Tel.: 0118 950 5950
www.chiropractic-uk.co.uk

British Homeopathy Association – We are the UK's leading homeopathic charity committed to the promotion and practice of homeopathy. We believe that homeopathy should be available to everyone. That's why we offer free and low cost appointments at our charitable clinics. Our aim is to build more awareness by promoting homeopathy and its practice, by funding reasearch and by ensuring that government, decision makers and healthcare professionals understand the benefits of homeopathy. We can provide information on homeopathy and qualified practitioners.

Address: CAN Mezzanine, 49-57 East Road, London, N1 6 AH
Tel.: 0203 640 5903
www.homeopathy-uk.org
They also have an online directory listing hundreds of registered homeopaths.
www.britishhomeopathic.org

British Medical Acupuncture Society – The BMAS is a registered charity established to stimulate and promote the use and scientific understading of acupuncture within medicine for the public benefit. If you want further information please do contact us. We have two offices (see below).

Address: BMAS London – Royal London Hospital for Integrated Medicine, 60 Great Ormond Street, London, WC1N 3HR
Tel.: 020 7713 9437
Address: BMAS Northwich – 2/3 Winnington Court, Northwich, Cheshire CW8 1AQ
Tel.: 01606 786 782
www.medical-acupuncture.co.uk

British Pain Society – The B.P.S. aims to promote education, training, research and development in all fields of pain. It endeavours to increase both professional and public awareness of the prevelance of pain and the facilities that are available for its management. The BPS is the oldest and largest multidisciplinary organisation in the field of pain within the UK. Chronic pain is suffered by over a third of the population in the UK.

Address: 3rd Floor Churchill House, 35 Red Lion Square, London, WC1R 4SG
email: info@britishpainsociety.org
Tel.: 020 7269 7840
www.britishpainsociety.org

British Register of Complemmentary Practitioners (BRCP) – It provides support and services for complemmentary therapy practitioners and shares information to inform and educate the public about Complemmentary Medicine. If you want to know about a local therapist or practitioner safe in the knowledge that they are qualified and insured, please do not hesitate to contact us.

Address: BRCP, P.O. Box 122, Wellington, TA21 1BX
Tel.: 0300 302 0715
www.brcp.uk

Centre for Pain Research (CPR) – We are a specialist research centre at Bath, made of academics, clinicians, researchers and students with a shared interest in pain and pain management.

For any enquiries contact: Dr. Lisa Austin, Research Hub Manager.
Address: 1 West Level 3, University of Bath, BA2 7AY.
E-mail: l.ausin@bath.ac.uk

General Osteopathic Council – The General Osteopathic Council regulates the practice of osteopaths in the UK. We can provide details of registered osteopaths near you, and a wide range of leaflets on back problems and how osteopathy can work. We work with the public and the osteopathic profession to promote patient safety by setting, maintaining and developing standards of osteopathic practice and conduct. By law, osteopaths must be registered with us to practice in the UK.

Address: Osteopathy House, 176 Tower Bridge Road, London, SE1 3LU
E-mail: gosc@osteopathy.org.uk
Tel.: 02073576655
www.osteopathy.org.uk

Institute for Complementary and Natural Medicine (ICNM) – The ICNM is a charity which provides the public with information about the safe and proper choice of Complementary Medicine. The ICNM offers a search facility for the public to access practitioners and therapists who are members of the BRCP (see above). The ICNM promotes and supports Best Practice for all practitioners and therapists who work with Complementary Medicine.

Address: 32-36 Loman Street, London, SE1 0EH
Tel.: 020 7922 7980
www.naturaltherapypages.co.uk/association/institute_of_complementary_medicine

---

Institute of Osteopathy – The iO is here to support, unite, develop and promote the osteopathy profession for the improvement of public health and patient care. Osteopaths use a wide range of gentle hands-on techniques that focus on releasing tension, improving mobility and optimising function. If you would like to find a local osteopath in your local area, do contact us.

Address: 3 Park Terrace, Manor Park, Luton LU1 3HN
Tel.: 01582 488 455
www.iosteopathy.org

Men's Health Forum – It is the charity's ambition that all men and boys, particularly those in the most disadvantaged areas and communities, will have the information, services and treatments they need to live healthier, longer and more fulfilling lives. We also do research and campaigning aiming to reduce the tragic deaths of men and boys who simply die too young of preventable health problems.

Address: 49-51 East Road, London N1 6AH
Tel.: 020 7922 7908
www.menshealthforum.org.uk

Pain Concern UK – We are a charity working to support and inform people with pain and those who care for them, whether family, friends or healthcare professionals. We provide a medical helpline and a listening-earphone service for people who want to talk over their pain problems. We are registered as a charity in Scotland, but have expanded our focus to work with pain clinics, medical specialists and volunteers from across the UK, and our membership also reflects this.

Their help service is accessible at: help@painconcern.org.uk
Address: 62-66 Newcraighall Road, Edinburgh EH15 3HS
General enquiries (email): info@painconcern.org.uk
Tel.: 0300 102 0162
Address: The Gateway, 85-101 Sankey Street, Warrington WA1 1SR
Tel.: 0300 102 0162
Helpline: 0300 123 0789
www.painconcern.org.uk

Pain Support – We offer support for all those with long-term pain lasting 6 months or more. Our website is packed full with pain relief techniques, tips, resources and advice. The Pain Support website will help you move forward in your life with better chronic pain self-management.

They have NO address and NO phone number, but they have a vast amount of information on line.
www.painsupport.co.uk

The **Alexander Technique Centre –** We teach one-to-one lessons and group classes. We also train Alexander Technique teachers and run professional development workshops for teachers and trainee teachers. We will provide information on teachers near you.

Address: 27 Blackfriars Road, London SE1 8NY
e-mail: info@alexandercentre.co.uk
Tel.: 0800 170 1357
www.alexandercentre.co.uk

The **Friends of the Alexander Technique –** It is a registered charity and is fully supported by the Society of Teachers of the Alexander Technique (STAT). Friends of the Alexander Technique is a participative organisation for people who use the Alexander Technique in any aspects of their lives. Our aim is to encourage a sense of community amongst people at all levels of experience in the Alexander Technique, with a view of providing support for those who are learning, living and teaching these ideas and to inspire others to become interested in them.

Address: STAT, P.O. Box 75989, London E11 9 GZ
e-mail: info@stat.org.uk
Tel.: 020 8885 6524
www.alexandertechnique.co.uk/no-section/friends-alexander-technique

---

The Pain Management Centre – It is internally recognised as a centre of excellence in patient care and research. Our area of interest include chronic pain conditions such as back pain, neck/shoulder pain, neuropathies and complex regional pain syndriome (CRPS). The aim of these studies is to improve our understanding of pain conditions and to establish new treatments for our patients.

Address: St. Thomas'Hospital, Westminster Bridge Road, London SE1 7EH
Tel.: 020 7188 7188
www.guysandstthomas.nhs.uk

The **Pain Relief Foundation –** We are a charity working to support and inform people with pain and those who care for them. We belief that pain is best faced together by the 'Pain Community' of people with pain, their family, supporters and healthcare professionals. We carry out reasearch leading to the alleviation of chronic pain and find improve methods of treating it. We also provide scientific education to health professionals.

Address: Clinical Sciense Centre, University Hospital Aintree, Lower Lane, Liverpool L9 7AL
Tel.: 0151 529 5820
www.painrelieffoundation.org.uk

Versus Arthritis – It was formed in 2018 following a merger of Arthritis Care and Arthritis Reaseach UK. Alongside volunteers, healthcare professionals, researchers and friends, we do everything we can to push back against arthritis. Our advisers aim to bring all the information and advice about arthritis into one place to provide tailored support for you.Together we will continue to develop break-through treatments, campaign relentlessly for arthritis to be seen as a priority, and to support each other whenever we need it.

Address: Copeman House, St. Mary's Court, St. Mary's Gate, Chesterfield S41 7TD
e-mail: enquiries@versusarthritis.org
Tel.: 0300 790 0400
www.versusarthritis.org

www.ingramcontent.com/pod-product-compliance
Ingram Content Group UK Ltd.
Pitfield, Milton Keynes, MK11 3LW, UK
UKHW020132250726
13967UKWH00002B/614